Eye Floaters – Vitreous Opacity or Light of Consciousness?

Floaters between Science and Religion, A challenge to Ophthalmology, Visual Nervous System, Migraine Aura

Floco Tausin
Leuchtstruktur Verlag

ISBN 9783907400906

Copyright © Leuchtstruktur Verlag / Floco Tausin 2022

Print:
kdp.amazon.com

Further information about the subject of eye floaters:
eye-floaters.info

Weitere Informationen zum Thema Mouches volantes:
mouches-volantes.com

Contents

Introduction
7

1. Floaters between Science and Religion
13

2. A Challenge to Ophthalmology
31

3. Do Eye Floaters Arise from the Visual Nervous System?
49

4. The Spiritual Dimension of the Migraine Aura
69

Author Floco Tausin
86

Introduction

In the mid-1990s I met a man named Nestor living in the solitude of the hilly Emmental region of Switzerland. Nestor has a unique and provocative claim: that he focuses for years on a constellation of huge shining spheres and strings which have been formed in his field of vision. He interprets this phenomenon as a subtle structure formed by our consciousness which in turn creates our material world. Nestor, who calls himself a seer, ascribes this subjective visual perception to his long lasting efforts to develop his consciousness. This includes an appropriate lifestyle as well as practices for both temporary and permanent increase of the intensity of consciousness. Nestor claims that, through these physical and concentrative practices, his spheres and strings that were at first small, far away and very mobile, had now enlarged, come closer, started to shine, and now he could hold them in suspension with his gaze. There, in the centre of the visual field, there would be one last sphere, the "source", into which we human beings would enter when we fall asleep or die. Nestor is convinced that if we get near this last sphere as much as possible in our lifetime, we have the chance to enter into it keeping our full consciousness – and thereby overcome death.

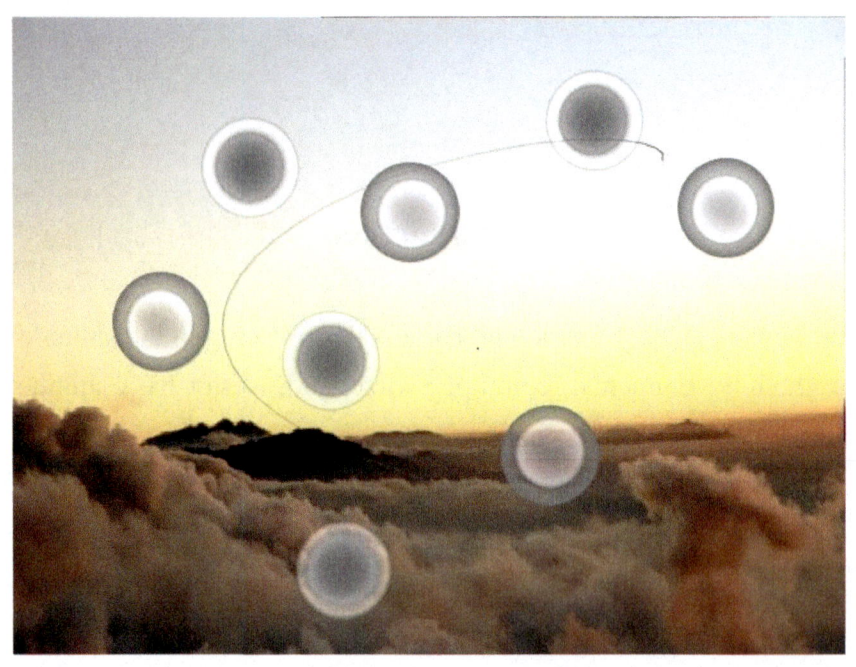

Core-surround floaters in a seer's view. Source: Floco Tausin.

Vitreous opacity or light of consciousness?

I have told the story of my apprenticeship with Nestor in my book *Mouches Volantes – Eye Floaters as Shining Structure of Consciousness* (2009). When I started seeing these dots and strings myself, I did a lot of research. I found out that this subjective visual phenomenon was not only known, but widespread. However, the way it is commonly understood deviates significantly from Nestor's statements. In our culture, the authority to interpret this phenomenon has been with ophthalmology for centuries. There, these dots and strands are known by the term "eye floaters" or *mouches volantes* (French for "flying flies"). Eye floaters are an entoptic appearance, i.e. caused by the human visual system itself. In that case, it's a cloudiness of the vitreous body that affects the patient's vision. This perception is explained by the fact that the vitreous body shrinks and liquefies with increasing age (*syneresis*). Parts of the vitreous structure consisting of hyaluronic acid and collagen fibrils clump together and cast shadows on the retina, which become visible as scattered mobile dots and strings. Eye floaters are considered harmless. The general medical advice is to ignore them. As a precaution, one may have their eyes examined for a possible retinal detachment. This is especially necessary when the floaters are suddenly accompanied by large dark clouds ("soot rain") and lightning.

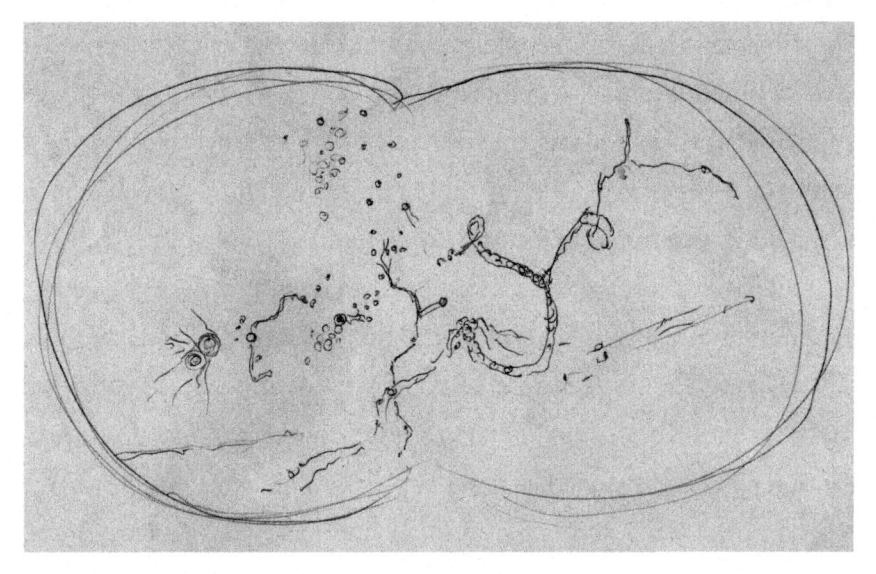

Common eye floaters. Source: Floco Tausin.

Many people can see their floaters if they pay attention. To most, they are just a curiosity and not really distracting. Some people, however, feel disturbed by their dots and strands, such that they are considering surgical measures. Vitrectomy, for example, removes parts of the vitreous humour. Laser vitreolysis, on the other hand, attempts to break up single floater strands through fast laser pulses. However, such treatments are risky and are not recommended by most ophthalmologists to remove the harmless eye floaters.

So, are eye floaters vitreous opacities, or are they the light of consciousness? Nestor has identified eye floaters as the first appearance of what he calls "shining structure" or "luminous spheres" and "luminous strings" and understands as the light of consciousness. If he is right, then the ophthalmological understanding of eye floaters would be completely wrong. How can that be? Fact is that ophthalmologists cannot always find the floaters in the eyes of their patients. This is not only true for looking into the eyes with a slit lamp, but also for more sophisticated methods such as ultrasound examination or optical coherence tomography (OCT). Why is it that not all eye floaters can be objectively located? Ophthalmologists assert that some floaters are just too small or too close to the retina to be detected. If this is the case, then the methods and devices available are not efficient enough until now. Another possibility is that there are different types of subjective visual phenomena summarized under the term "eye floaters", and that one of them is not a vitreous opacity. Even if actual vitreous opacities and the first appearances of the shining structure look similar at first glance, there are clear differences on closer inspection. The former are rather described and depicted as something dark and blurred, like shadows, streaks or spots. The latter, on the other hand, are scattered transparent or luminous dots and strands with clear contours. The dots contain a core, and the strands are filled with dots. The former can be detected and treated, the latter cannot – simply because they are no vitreous opacities. But what are they then?

This book is dedicated to this question. All of the texts have been published before and revised. In the first chapter, *Floaters between Science and Religion*, I consider the meaning of the subtle characteristics of eye floaters, as conveyed by Nestor. Suggesting that floaters can be relevant not only for individual spirituality, but for society and ophthalmology as well, I address the following questions: how do floaters relate to entoptic phenomena which are known to have spiritual relevance in some indigenous shamanic societies? Do Nestor's claims about floaters require a modified ophthalmological interpretation? And to what extent is it reasonable to think of floaters as a spiritual phenomenon? Then, in *A Challenge to Ophthalmology*, I discuss one of these questions in more detail: do we need a new physiological understanding of eye floaters? As I will show, a careful observation of floaters reveals properties that challenge the dominant view and call for a reconsideration of the ophthalmological explanation. The third chapter, *Do Eye Floaters Arise from the Visual Nervous System?*, tries to provide an alternative physiological approach to eye floaters. These structures strikingly resemble the morphological and functional structures of receptive fields of the visual nervous system. Thus the hypothesis of this article: so-called "idiopathic" (harmless) eye floaters are a visible expression of neuronal processes. As in the case of other entoptic phenomena like phosphenes or form constants, the neurological explanation of floaters is suitable to bridge the gap between science and spirituality. The final chapter, *The Spiritual Dimension of the Migraine Aura*, can be understood as an application of the results in the previous chapters. It deals with an alternative and spiritual approach to the common migraine headache. The starting point are the entoptic phenomena – eye floaters among others – which appear during the migraine aura. These phenomena make migraine headaches, like shamanic trance, seem to be an intensification of consciousness, with the exception that the psychophysical system of the migraine patient is not able to handle that state. Accordingly, exercises and life styles are suggested that are used in spiritual traditions to strengthen body and consciousness, and to regulate the flow of energy.

1
Floaters between Science and Religion

First published:
Tausin, Floco (2011): "The Eye Floater Phenomenon". *Edgescience* 6: 14-17

In history of religion and art, a multitude of cases are known in which spiritually committed individuals report about abstract or figurative subjective visual phenomena they experienced – often while in ritually induced altered states of consciousness (cf. Tausin 2010b; Müller-Ebeling 1993). Usually, these phenomena are interpreted in terms of the cultural and religious tradition of the individual. One of these individuals is Nestor, a seer from the Swiss Emmental who claims to concentrate on an entoptic phenomenon known as "eye floaters". His case, though, seems to be exceptional in two regards: first, Nestor himself is aware of, and considers, the ophthalmological explanation of floaters. And second, floaters are a common and wide spread phenomenon, experienced by a lot of people who do not claim to live a particularly religious or spiritual life.

In the course of a learning time with Nestor, I tried to understand the phenomenon from an ophthalmological point of view, as well as from my own observations. My objective was to comprehend Nestor's claims about the spiritual relevance of this phenomenon (Tausin, 2009a). In this article I will address the following questions that I have been considering in the process:

1) What are floaters?
2) What makes Nestor think of floaters as a spiritual phenomenon?
3) Are there any equivalents in the history of science and religion to understanding floaters in terms of spiritually relevant visionary experiences?
4) Does Nestor's claim require a new ophthalmological understanding of eye floaters, and how so?
5) Is it reasonable to think of floaters as a spiritual phenomenon, and to what extent?

Eye floaters in ophthalmology

"Eye floaters" (*mouches volantes* in French and German ophthalmology) is a collective term used in ophthalmology for all possible opacities in the vitreous body. Many of them can be traced to physiological disorders like retinal detachment, diabetic vitreoretinopathy, as well as Marfan's, Ehlers-Danlos, and Stickler's syndromes.

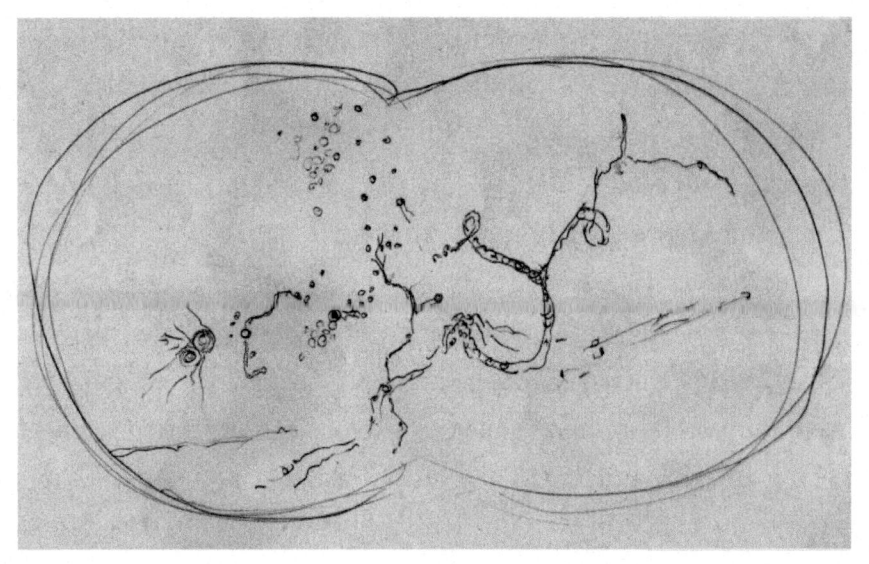

'Idiopathic' eye floaters in the visual field. Source: Floco Tausin.

The floaters at issue, though – which are also the most experienced floater type – are considered as 'idiopathic', i.e. without pathological cause. They are seen as mobile and scattered semi-transparent dots and strands in the visual field, best perceived in bright light conditions. These dots and strands float according to the eye movements which makes them hard to focus on. The explanations vary between remaining embryonic stem cells, cell debris between the retina and the vitreous humour, and hyaluronic vitreous fibrils clumped together due to vitreous liquefaction and posterior vitreous detachment (Trick 2007; Sendrowski/Bronstein 2010).

Nestor's teaching: the structure of consciousness and the inner sense

Nestor's statements about eye floaters differ significantly from the ophthalmologic explanation (cf. Tausin 2010a, 2009a). According to him, these spheres and strings emerged from consciousness. They form a coherent structure on which we project our material world like on a screen. They are directly connected with our will. And ultimately, our pure egoless consciousness fits into one single sphere in this structure. For Nestor, we see these spheres and strings not with our eyes but with an "inner sense" or the "third eye". He characterizes this inner sense as an eye that gradually opens up through the withdrawal of the external senses as experienced in concentration exercises. Therefore, he explains the initial symptoms of floaters as an indication of the third eye beginning to open. The fact that many people see floaters in our contemporary Western societies means, according to Nestor, that many people already have a connection to their inner sense, even if they don't work with it consciously. Any activity that increases attentiveness of a human being is understood by Nestor as "spiritual" in nature.

With such statements, Nestor ascribes an extraordinary meaning to the visual phenomena called "floaters": they are a spiritual phenomenon, and thus a directly perceptible starting point for our own spiritual development, for the realization of our "true selves". But what made Nestor utter such claims? According to him, he deduces these propositions from his own seeing. It is important to understand that his description of the spheres and strings differs from the one of other people. He doesn't see scattered small dots and strings that drift away permanently, but large, bright spheres and tubes which he is able to hold in suspension and, therefore, to see clearly. His claim to deal with what is commonly called "floaters" is based on his experience of a transformation, resulting from a specific lifestyle, including an ethical attitude, a natural and balanced diet, a combination of physical and breathing exercises inspired from yogic practices, as well as concentration and meditation practices. Long and short term effects of such practices lead to altered states of consciousness that change visual perception. To be more precise, Nestor pleads to have observed the "lighting up" and "zooming in" of floaters: former transparent tiny dots and strands are now seen as large spheres and tubes full of light.

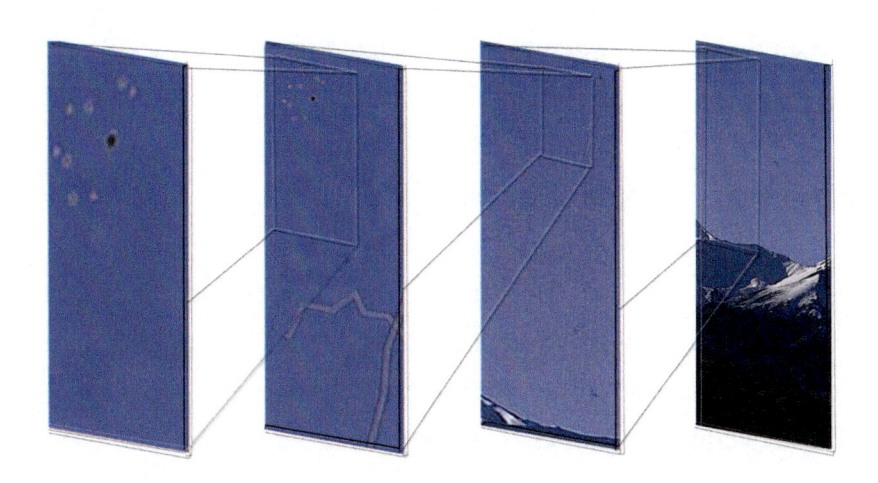

The zoom effect of shining structure floaters. Source: Floco Tausin.

The whole process is goal-oriented: the "zooming in" is experienced as a forward movement within this "shining structure" of floaters. This means that a seer, gradually or abruptly, focuses on new spheres that appear in the upper and rear part of the visual field. Nestor calls this visual forward movement "the path in the shining structure". This path is not only a path of intensification and progression, but also a path of reduction: in the beginning, Nestor experienced seeing a large quantity of tiny dots and strings which moved before his eyes without any recognizable order or obvious meaning – this is what people usually call "floaters". Today, he speaks of a single huge sphere at the end of that way, the "navel", which he is drawn to, and into which he believes he will enter to become one with the structure, experiencing a state of bliss. Nestor's path is thus a mystical path: he believes that we lost the primordial unity with the "picture" in the process of embodiment and of becoming individual and separate personalities. The way in the shining structure leads back to this unity.

Floaters and entoptic phenomena

In the past 150 years, modern science has provided concepts to understand the physiological aspects of at least some of the extraordinary subjective visual phenomena. For example, many of the abstract geometric figures in indigenous art or in shamans' or yogis' ritually induced visions can be understood as "entoptic phenomena" (cf. Thurston 1997). Entoptic phenomena are coloured or bright moving geometric shapes and patterns in the visual field, caused by certain conditions of the human visual nervous system. In the 19th century, European and American opticians and physiologists developed a broad interest in entoptic phenomena. To generate and study entoptics, they conducted experiments by stimulating brain and retina, electrically at first, later also with mind-altering substances. Especially in the 1960s and 70s, a number of experiments on subjects were conducted using agents such as THC, mescaline, psilocybin and LSD. A worldwide ban on these substances interrupted the drug based research on entoptics (cf. Tausin 2010c).

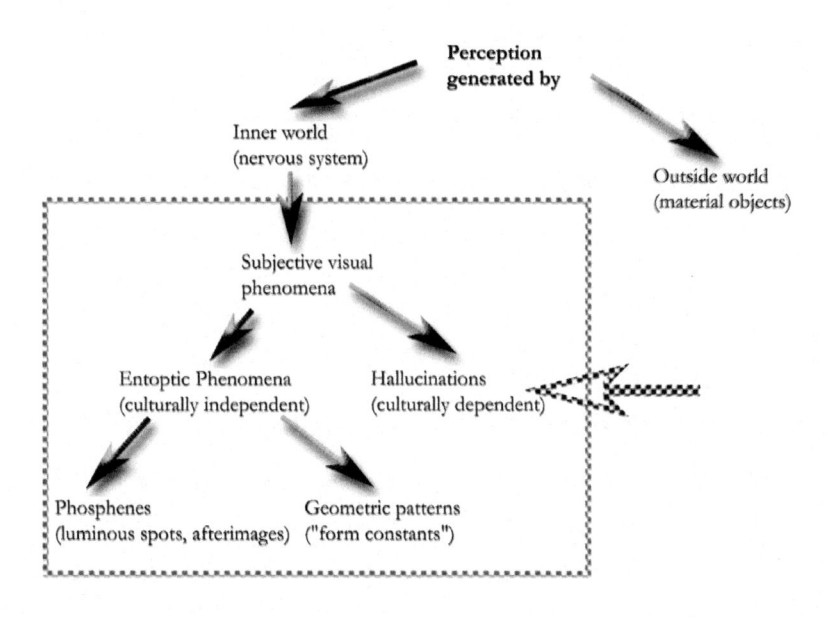

Types of subjective visual phenomena. Source: Floco Tausin.

In the second half of the 20th century, some scholars of anthropology and archaeology referred to this heritage of research to explain abstract geometric signs often depicted in the art of shamanic indigenous societies. For example, the anthropologist Gerardo Reichel-Dolmatoff (1975, 1978, 1987, 1997) conducted field research among the Tukano Indians of the Eastern Vaupés (Colombia). The Tukano shamans use hallucinogens like Banisteriopsis (*yagé/yajé, ayahuasca, caapi*) in divinatory and medical rituals. The visions of geometric figures like circles, dots, lines, curves, zigzag lines, grids etc., appearing in an initial phase of the visionary experience, are identified by the Tukanos with cosmological, mythological and social concepts and serve as an inspiration for their art. Reichel-Dolmatoff explains these signs as "phosphenes", induced by the hallucinogens (cf. Tausin 2010b).

Another example is the archaeological controversy about a neuropsychological interpretation of the rock and cave art of the later Palaeolithic (about 40'000 to 10'000 BC). Ever since the discovery of the European Palaeolithic caves, archaeologists have been wondering about the importance and meaning of such geometric representations, accompanying the vivid depictions of animals. In 1988, David Lewis-Williams and Thomas Dowson brought forward the original thesis that Palaeolithic art is inspired by entoptic phenomena (or, more specifically, "form constants"), seen and depicted by shamans or spiritual men and women during altered states of consciousness. Entoptic phenomena fit in their line of thinking, for they are said to be culturally independent, generated by states of the visual nervous system only – which makes them comparable to figures in modern shamanic art in order to support the thesis (Lewis-Williams/Dowson 1988; cf. Tausin 2010).

Similar patterns of entoptic phenomena in different times and cultures. Source: Lewis-Williams/Dowson 1988.

Towards a new ophthalmological interpretation of eye floaters

Thus, while scholars do acknowledge that the visual experience of so-called entoptic phenomena can have a cultural or spiritual relevance to their observers under certain conditions, eye floaters are tacitly excluded from this line of thinking. In my opinion, there are two main reasons for this: first, eye floaters are an ordinary phenomenon, perceived by a lot of people in everyday consciousness. And second, floaters are explained as idiopathic opacities in the vitreous body, i.e. "entophthalmic" rather than "entoptic" phenomena – eye rubbish, so to speak. Both reasons seem to mock the idea that they could have a positive, spiritual meaning to any rational being. However, I would like to reconsider these points drawing on Nestor's and my own visual experience with floaters.

First, while eye floaters do show up in ordinary consciousness states, they also constantly look different – which is, in my opinion, pointing to the fact that there is no "ordinary", but a constantly changing consciousness. Anybody taking the time to carefully observe her or his floaters recognizes that they constantly change size, brightness, and velocity. A closer inspection reveals that this alteration depends on a number of factors, some of which are outer conditions like the brightness and colour of the background against which floaters are viewed. Others may be called "inner" or "psychic" conditions, like attention span, mood, degree of concentration, stress and the like. It's not by accident that vision improvement schools propose to influence floaters through relaxation practices – in order to get rid of them, though (Tausin 2009b). As I have demonstrated above, Nestor is making the same claim, differing only in the degree of psychophysical abilities like concentration, calmness, "energy metabolism" etc. Thus, it is perfectly conceivable that a human's perception of floaters could change to the extent explained above, revealing certain features that are experienced as "meaningful" or "spiritual", like the "path in the shining structure", or the "navel".

Second, today's academic ophthalmology provides a sensible explanation of floaters as "vitreous opacities". Considering the variegated history of ophthalmological "meaning making" and objectification of this highly subjective phenomenon (Plange 1990), this has never been an easy task. In my opinion, there is no reason to accept today's ophthalmology's explanation for it still fails to explain some of the more subtle floater characteristics that can be revealed through careful observation (cf. Tausin 2009d). For example, the morphological regularity of eye floaters: floater spheres are perfectly circular and concentric and show a core and a surround. Two contrasting types of spheres can be distinguished: such with bright surrounds and dark core, and such with dark surrounds and bright core. It is questionable if this morphological regularity really represents hyaluronic fibrils or cells clumped together. Or, the change of the size of the spheres and strings: the very same sphere may appear big and diffuse or small and focused. The transition of one state to another is fluent and a matter of minutes or even seconds. For the sake of simplicity I distinguish between a "relaxed" (big) state and a "concentrated" (small) state. Generally, it seems as if most eye floaters were, at first, relaxed and thus bigger, nearer, and more transparent. With increasing time of observation, however, they change into a concentrated state. After abandoning concentration, this latter state of the spheres and strands will change into the state of relaxation again – a quick glance to somewhere else may suffice.

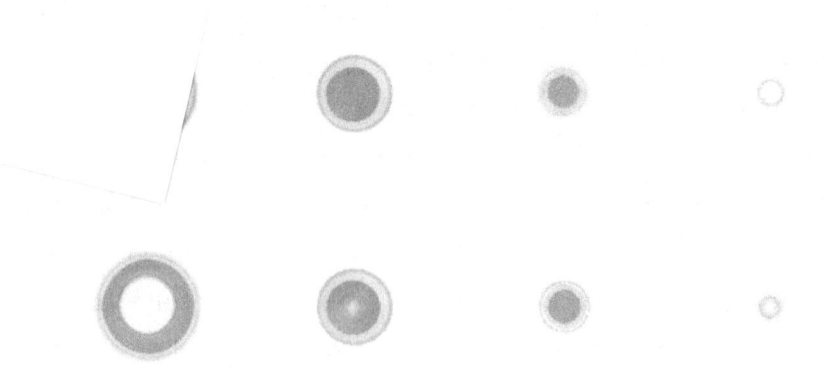

The two types of floaters spheres in a relaxed (left) and concentrated (right) state. Source: Floco Tausin.

Eye debris, in contrast, is not supposed to change size in that regular manner. Nor is it supposed to light up, to give yet another example, like floaters do in the process of concentration. Also, the sinking of the dots and strands is worth considering: eye floaters react sensitive to eye movements. It seems as if they would always move in the direction in which we look. But as soon as we keep the eyes still and observe the floaters from the angle of vision, we recognize that they sink – sometimes faster, sometimes slower. This sinking may be taken as evidence for the debris nature of floaters, debris floating in the vitreous humour and sinking due to the force of gravity. However, this argument is disqualified if we recall that the image of the visual world on the retina is inverted – which means that any sinking down of floaters as seen by the observer would require the corresponding particles in the vitreous to ascend. In this case, too, careful observation reveals that the sinking rather seems to be related to the consciousness state, viz. it tends to slow down in states in which floaters are seen big and shiny. A further indication of the limits of the ophthalmological explanation is found in the everyday practice of eye doctors who vainly try to find the floater type at issue in the patients' eyes (cf. Tausin 2009c).

All of this suggests that the type of floaters at discussion should be reconsidered by ophthalmology or physiology. With the concepts at hand, and based on my subjective experiences and experiments with floaters, I strongly suspect them to be an "entoptic" rather than "entophthalmic" phenomena. In other words, I suggest that they are related or generated by the visual nervous system (Tausin 2009d).

Conclusions

Subjective visual phenomena have been significant for many societies throughout history. They have been observed, recorded and interpreted by spiritual women and men over and over. This way, such phenomena entered into particular cultures, as a source of inspiration for artists, philosophers and religious thinkers and believers alike. Scientific evidence suggests that many of these visionary experiences correlate with entoptic phenomena. This fits well with our thinking influenced to a large extent by cognitive and neurosciences and their reductionist view on religious experiences as "particular brain states". Eye floaters, on the other hand, are perceived as a "particular vitreous state" which seems to exclude any relationship to "spirituality". Careful observations of floaters, however, reveal that psychic factors change the appearance of floaters – pointing to their "entoptic" nature.

Yet, does this also indicate a "spiritual" nature of floaters? As is the case with entoptics, it depends on the definition of "spirituality". The case of Nestor demonstrates that floaters, too, can have an extraordinary meaning for human beings, expressed in terms of religion and spirituality. For most Western people, however, it has not. The question, therefore, is: what do we gain by a spiritual interpretation of floaters? To me, this interpretation has, under specific conditions, positive effects in individuals and society: on the one hand, for individuals who suffer from the floater type under discussion, this interpretation may serve as an alternative coping strategy completing academic ophthalmological and psychological treatment. Individuals dedicated to "know thyself" or consciousness development, on the other hand, take floaters (and other entoptic phenomena) as meditation object and feedback system for psychophysical practices. A 'floaters spirituality' is, in my opinion, a rather rational spirituality, based on sensual perception, research and experiment. Scrutinizing one's own floaters in this context could contribute to improve or modify the scientific understanding of floaters. This, in turn, helps to bridge gaps between science and religion, which is, in my opinion, an imperative in an age in which the negative effects of a one-sided focusing on the assumptions of materialistic philosophy – often promoting isolation and irresponsibility – are evident.

Many people have recognized the problems and orient themselves to new intellectual and spiritual values. The visual path conveyed by consciousness researchers of past and present societies is a possible approach to literally reconcile the "spiritual" and the "material", or, as Nestor puts it, the "inner screen" and the "outer screen". To me, the mobile dots and strands called "eye floaters" are a particularly suitable meditation object. Unlike other entoptic phenomena, floaters are visible in our everyday states of consciousness, and we can move them in our visual field anytime. We can play with them at will, concentrate and meditate on them, and observe and try to verify claims about them, made by friends, ophthalmologists or seers like Nestor.

References

Lewis-Williams, J. D.; Dowson, T. A. (1988): "The Signs of All Times: Entoptic Phenomena in Upper Paleolithic Art". *Current Anthropology 29*, no. 2: 201-245

Müller-Ebeling, Claudia (1993): "Visionäre Kunst". Welten des Bewusstseins (*Vol. 1: Ein interdisziplinärer Dialog)*, ed. by Adolf Dittrich, Albert Hofmann et al. Berlin

Plange, Hubertus (1990): "Muscae volitantes – von frühen Beobachtungen zu Purkinjes Erklärung". *Gesnerus 47*: 31-44

Reichel-Dolmatoff, Gerardo (1975): *The Shaman and the Jaguar. A Study of Narcotic Drugs Among the Indians of Colombia.* Philadelphia: Temple University Press

Reichel-Dolmatoff, Gerardo (1978): *Beyond the Milky Way. Hallucinatory Imagery of the Tukano Indians.* Los Angeles: University of California

Reichel-Dolmatoff, Gerardo (1987): "Shamanism and art of the eastern Tukanoan Indians". *Iconography of Religions IX*, ed. by Th. P. van Baaren et al. Leiden u.a.: Brill

Reichel-Dolmatoff, Gerardo (1997): *Rainforest Shamans. Essays on the Tukano Indians of the Northwest Amazon.* Themis Books

Sendrowski, David P.; Bronstein, Mark A. (2010). "Current treatment for vitreous floaters". *Optometry 81:* 157-161

Tausin, Floco (2010a): "Eye Floaters. Floating spheres and strings in a seer's view". *Holistic Vision 2.* eye-floaters.info/news/news-june2010.htm#1 (11.9.22)

Tausin, Floco (2010b): "Lichter in der Anderswelt. Mouches volantes in der darstellenden Kunst moderner Schamanen". *Ganzheitlich Sehen 2/10.* mouches-volantes.com/news/newsjuni2010.htm#1 (11.9.22)

Tausin, Floco (2010c): "Entoptic phenomena as universal trance phenomena". *Soulful Living.* soulfulliving.com/entoptic-phenomena.htm (11.9.22)

Tausin, Floco (2009a): *Mouches Volantes. Eye Floaters as Shining Structure of Consciousness.* Bern: Leuchtstruktur Verlag

Tausin, Floco (2009b): "Sanftes Fliegenmittel. Mouches volantes in der alternativen Augenheilkunde". *Virtuelles Magazin 2000 53*. archiv.vm2000.net/53/FlocoTausin/FlocoTausin.html (11.9.22)

Tausin, Floco (2009c): "Mouches volantes nicht im Glaskörper?" *Ganzheitlich Sehen 4*. mouches-volantes.com/news/newsdezember2009.htm#2 (11.9.22)

Tausin, Floco (2009d): "Mouches volantes – Glaskörpertrübung oder Nervensystem?" *ExtremNews*, 22.12.09. extremnews.com/berichte/gesundheit/e01c12cc1d3c89f (11.9.22)

Thurston, Linda (1991): Entoptic Imagery in People and Their Art (M.A. thesis, 1991, *web edition 1997*). home.comcast.net/~markk2000/thurston/thesis.html (2011)

Trick, Gary L.; Kronenberg, Alaina (2007): "Entoptic Imagery and Afterimages". *Duane's Ophthalmology*, ed. by William Tasman and Edward A. Jaeger. Philadelphia: Lippincott Williams & Wilkins

2
A Challenge to Ophthalmology

First published:
Tausin, Floco (2011): "In-depth observations on eye floaters – A challenge to ophthalmology". Source: Link[1].

In ophthalmology, "eye floaters" is a collective term for vitreous opacities which are attributed to different causes. In most cases, however, the phenomenon is considered an 'idiopathic', i.e. non-pathological age-related cloudiness of the vitreous humour. In this article, my statements on floaters refer to this idiopathic type. According to ophthalmologists, this wide-spread symptom occurs due to the liquefaction (*synchysis*) and collapse of the collagen-hyaluronic structure of the vitreous humour (*syneresis*), which at some stage causes the detachment of the vitreous body from the retina (posterior vitreous detachment, PVD) (Sendrowski 2010). In daylight, vitreous structures that are clumped together cast shadows on the retina and become visible in the field of vision. Supposedly, this is what we see when we are looking at our mobile, scattered and transparent dots and strings.

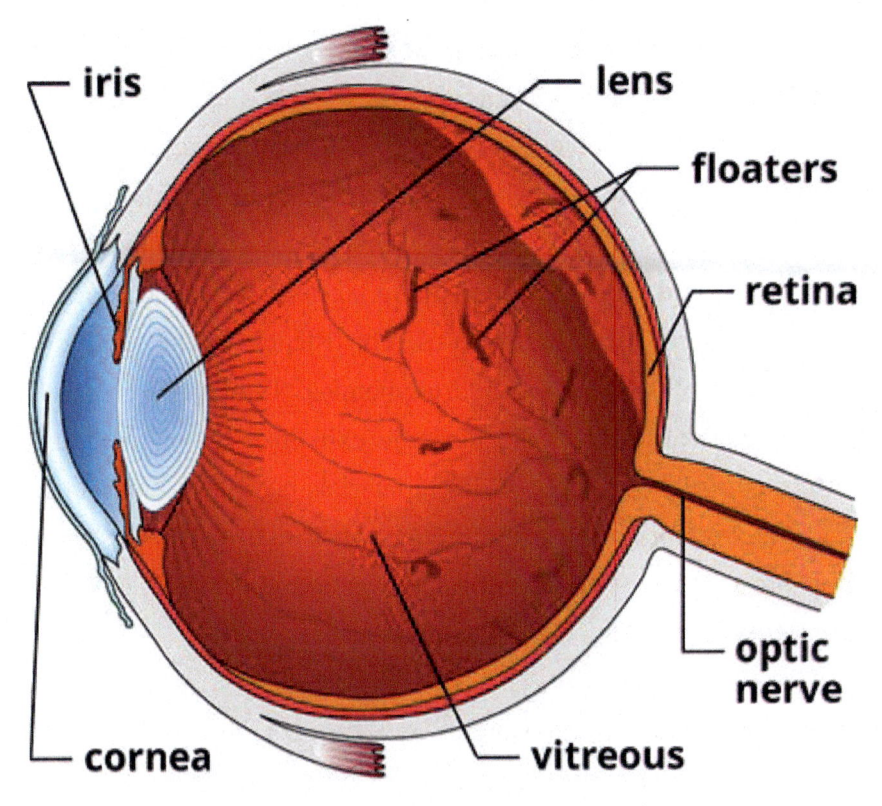

Floaters as harmless vitreous opacities. Source: Link[2].

This ophthalmological description is the latest offshoot in a tradition recorded since the time of Hippocrates. Over the centuries, the terms *konopia* (Greek, "midge"), *myio-eide* (Greek, "fly-like") and *muscae volitantes* (Latin, "flying flies") were used in Greek, Arab and Western European ophthalmology to describe subjective visual phenomena that look similar to flying flies (cf. Tausin 2018). From the beginning, a number of eye diseases and disorders were associated with flying flies, e.g. scotoma, cataract or retinal detachment. This reflects the endeavour to localize and explain eye floaters which, in turn, depends on the dominant philosophy: the ancient natural philosophers and scholars stressed that floaters must be in the liquids near the eye's lens, which was taken as the main element of seeing. Later, the materialistic-mechanical philosophy, on which early modern ophthalmology is based, promoted the notion of floaters as physical objects that move in the liquid of the vitreous humour near the retina, depending on the movement of the eyes, consistency of the medium, gravity as well as laws of hydrodynamics. 19th century Czech physiologist Jan Evangelista Purkinje explained the spheres and strings as fibrillae, vessels or dead materials near the retina whose shadows were projected on the retina when light enters the eyes. Most present-day eye doctors basically refer to Purkinje's description (Hirschberg 1889-1912; Plange 1990).

In my view, equating the spheres and strings with fly-like visual disorders or cloudiness is the result of a one-sided objective approach and of disciplinary narrowness. To balance this, I'm going to provide some challenging observations on floaters that I have collected in my many years of holistic research (Tausin 2009a, 2010b). Since individual observation is my starting point and base for my conclusions, I do not claim general validity, but I do encourage the inclined reader to spend some time in close observation of his or her own floaters – as a way to make my findings comprehensible.

Inconvenient questions to ophthalmology

Where does the morphological regularity of floaters come from?

Floaters are dots and strings. The strings are filled with rows of dots or spheres that are more or less clearly visible. The dots are circular and concentric. They contain a core and a surround, viz. they are polar. The polarity is joined by a dualism, for there are two types of dots: those with a bright surround and a dark core, and those with a dark surround and a bright core. So we can speak of a dualistic-polar principle in eye floaters. It's hard to imagine that randomly clumped vitreous fibrils produce dots with such clear and repeated morphological characteristics.

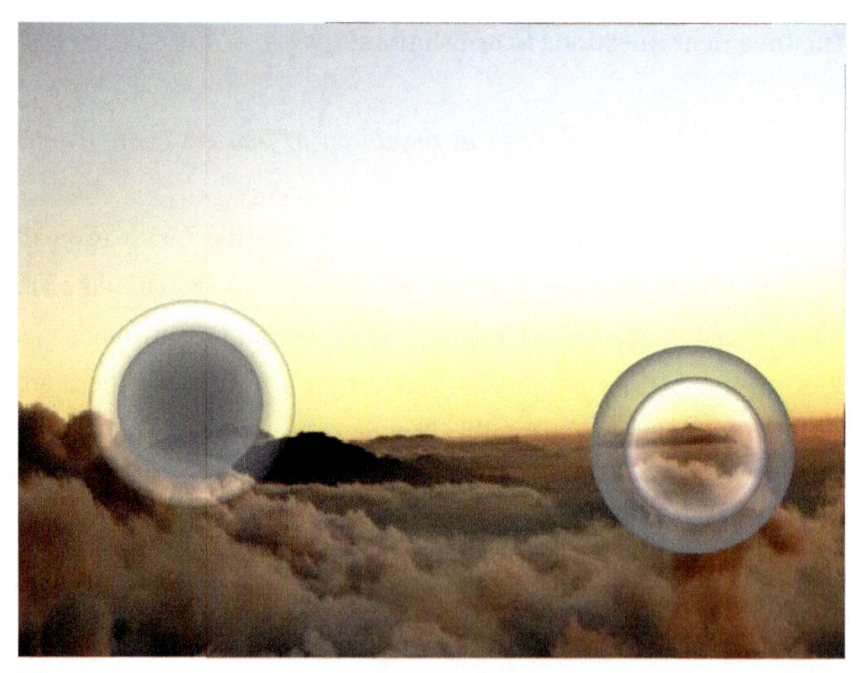

The two contrasting types of polar floater spheres. Source: Floco Tausin.

Why are there different states of floaters?

On closer observation, floater spheres and strings show different states over time: one and the same sphere can appear as big and rather hazy or as small and clearly outlined. The transition from one state to another is fluid and proceeds in different time duration. For the sake of simplicity, I distinguish an initial or relaxed state and a final or concentrated state. In general, it seems that most floaters are initially relaxed, viz. bigger, closer and more transparent. With increasing time of observation, they change into the concentrated state. After completion of the concentration – a quick glance to somewhere else may suffice –, the spheres and strings change back into the initial relaxed state.

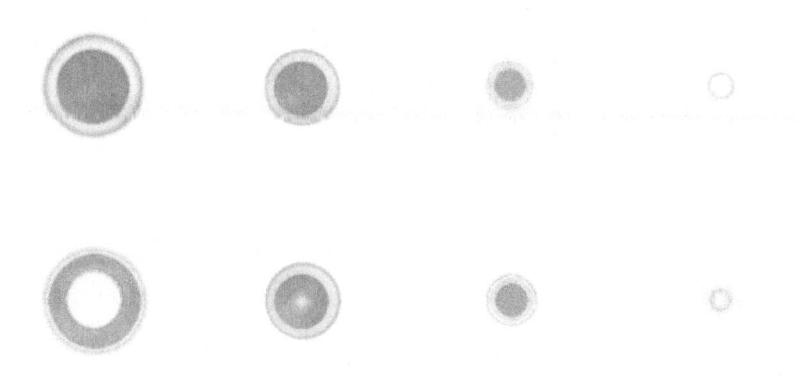

The two kinds of floater spheres in transition from a relaxed (left) to a concentrated (right) state. Source: Floco Tausin.

Why do floaters start to light up after some time of concentrated observation?

It is interesting to realize that, in the concentrated state, the spheres and strings increase in brilliance. Considering an energetic explanation for this, we could say that the amount of light or energy contained in a sphere or string does not change in the process of concentration. Rather, the energy gets compressed due to the reduction of space resulting in more brilliance (Tausin 2009a, 2010b). This effect may be influenced by "external" factors: it is encouraged by bright lighting conditions and the distance of the focal point – the closer the focal point, the brighter the floaters.

35

Also, observing the spheres and strings through the eyelashes or a pinhole in a sheet of paper lets the floaters appear concentrated. It is important to experience, though, that the concentration state is also reached without these aids, solely by focusing on floaters for a while. It is quickly brought to an end by visual distraction. Thus, floaters seem to reflect both outer and inner conditions of light and nearness, or concentration and presence, respectively.

Ophthalmology does not provide an explanation for the different states and the lighting up. Eye doctors, when asked, tend to ignore the question. Some try to explain the change in size as a result of floaters getting closer to the retina while looking up to the sky – gravity pulls the floaters back to the retina. The argument is unconvincing since the same effect can be observed irrespective of whether the eyes look up to the sky or down to the ground. Others trace the brilliance effect back to the scattering and reflectance of light. This is supposed to happen when light strikes the floaters inside the vitreous body (Tausin 2005a). The lens effect explanation implies the above-mentioned moving of floaters inside the vitreous humour. It is problematic insofar as it does not take into consideration the evident regularity of the altering of floater states (the nearer the focal point, the brighter the floaters; the longer the observation, the brighter the floaters). Moreover, the notion of moving dots and strings inside the vitreous body raises further questions.

Why do floaters move so quickly if the vitreous humour is a jelly-like fluid?

Floaters can be set in motion by eye movements. Doing so, they often seem to glide very easily and with high speed across the visual field. This is all the more surprising if we consider that the vitreous humour is thicker than water and described as a gel (Ruby 2007). How can there be any particles moving so quickly and effortlessly in a jelly-like mass? The classic answer is that the vitreous body liquefies over time and floaters become very mobile. But this leads straight to the next question.

If floaters are particles floating in liquefied parts of the vitreous body, why do we keep seeing the same spheres and strings?

Anyone who closely watches his or her floaters will soon become acquainted with them. For these spheres and strings remain the same for years. Through vigorous eye movements we may change the relative positions of the spheres and strings to one another, but only temporarily – the floaters take their starting position soon again. This observation contradicts the notion of free floating particles in the liquefied parts of the vitreous body – these would be whirled around with every eye movement and take up new constellations. The medical argument goes that some floaters do not move freely in the vitreous humour but are attached to the still existing vitreous structure. From the individual observer's perspective, there is no evidence: while some of the strands whose ends go beyond my visual field might be attached, other strings and all of the spheres do not seem to be attached anywhere – but still appear in their characteristic constellations.

Why do floaters tend to sink?

Through eye movements, we can move floaters in all directions. But as soon as we keep our eyes still, we realize that they sink down in our visual field – the nearer and bigger ones faster, the others more slowly. Gravity effects seem to be a plausible explanation for this sinking of physical particles in the vitreous body. The case is more complicated, though: As we know, our eyes project an upside-down image on the retina of what we are looking at in the world.

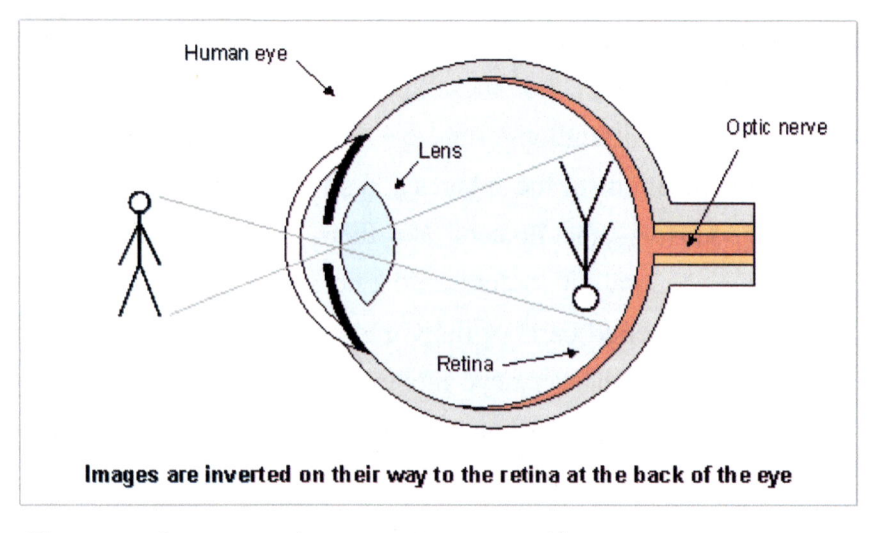

The inverted image on the retina. Source: Link[3].

If floaters were particles close to the retina that are pulled down by gravity and cast shadows on the retina, then I would have to see floaters rise in my visual field. Since I do not see floaters rising but sinking, the conclusion would be that the corresponding particles in the vitreous humour do not sink but rise. If that is true, there would be other forces than gravity influencing the upward movement of floaters.

I have asked dozens of eye doctors about this with no convincing results. Most ignore the fact of the inverted retinal image, or consider floaters or the retinal image isolated from one another. Some admit that floaters have to rise in the vitreous body if we see them sinking in our visual field. This leads them to speculate about thermodynamics or density as responsible mechanisms for that observation: according to this, eye floaters could be transported upwards by the convection flow. Physically, such flows arise, for example, when a heat source produces differences in temperature and thus in densities of a liquid. But whether the natural heat effect is really sufficient to produce significant currents in the vitreous humour is rather questionable. For example, it requires an artificial heat source to produce convection flows strong enough to transport medicinal substances through the vitreous humour (Narasimhan et al., 2015, 2013). In addition, if eye floaters were moved by convection currents, they would not only rise, but sink again as the humour cools down in the upper part of the vitreous body. This means that we would have to see our floaters first sink down, then rise up – without moving our eyes. According to my observation though, floaters only rise when I look up (cf. Tausin 2010a).

Further inconsistencies in ophthalmology

Why can't eye doctors see floaters in the eyes?

If the so-called "idiopathic eye floaters" really are clouding particles in the vitreous body, then one would think that eye doctors are able to see them when scanning the patients' eyes with devices like slit lamps, ultrasound imaging or optical coherence tomography (OCT). In reality, there is often a discrepancy between the patient's observation of eye floaters and the doctor's findings in the eye. In many cases, doctors can't see anything while patients very clearly perceive, describe and draw their eye floaters (cf. Weber-Varszegi et al. 2008; Tausin 2008). Then the diagnosis goes somewhat like "age-related harmless eye floaters", together with the advice to just ignore them. Explanations for this discrepancy are easily found: the opacities are too small to be relevant; the technology used is not accurate enough; the doctors do a poor examining job; the patient is exaggerating or has a mental problem. While there might be some truth in all these points, we also should keep in mind the possibility that floaters are not what ophthalmology claims.

It is no surprise that explanatory innovation comes from laser surgeons. In order to treat floaters with the Nd-YAG laser, surgeons have to localize and recognize the different floater types very carefully. The eye doctors James Johnson and Scott Geller explain on their websites that some floaters, especially those in young people, cannot be seen and treated with laser. The description of these "ill-defined" floaters fits the idiopathic ones at issue. The surgeons hold the opinion that this type is not located in the vitreous body, but must be between vitreous body and retina, a space called *bursa premacularis* (Geller n/a; Johnson n/a; cf. Tausin 2009b). This space is potential insofar as it exists only if fluids separate the vitreous body from the retina. In these fluids, rests of cells or fibrils could remain that become visible as floaters. While the theory is not acknowledged among eye doctors – as laser surgery of floaters is itself treated with reservation by many –, it does not contradict the main strategy to remove floaters: vitrectomy.

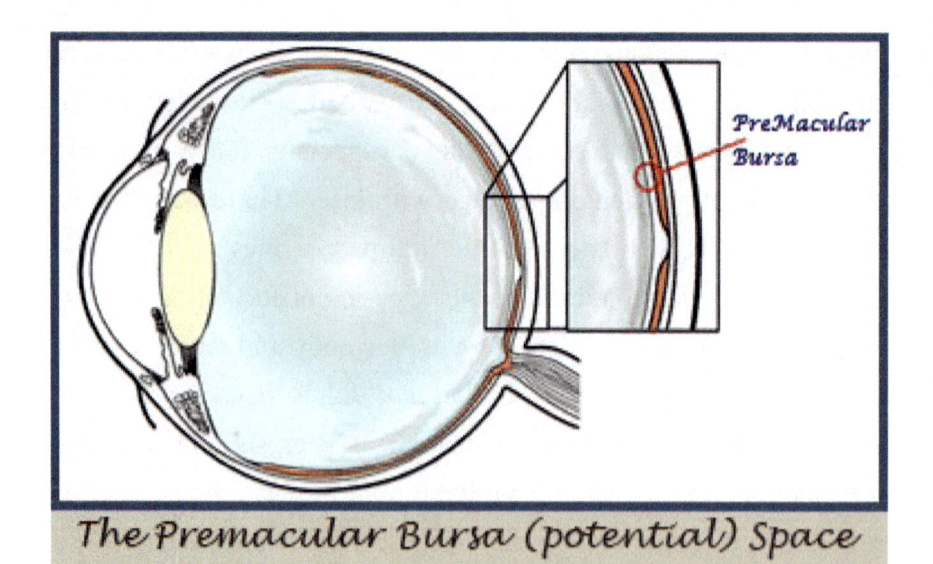

The premacular bursa as a potential space for non-detectable and non-treatable eye floaters. Source: Link[4].

Does vitrectomy prove the vitreous opacity theory of floaters?

The most powerful argument for the notion of floaters as vitreous opacities are the different forms of vitrectomy, a surgery to remove and replace the whole or parts of the vitreous humour. Laser surgeons assume that even bursa floaters might be removed by vitrectomy if the vitreous body is previously detached from the retina (cf. Tausin 2009b). In literature, there are cases of successful floaters-only vitrectomies (FOV), or "floaterectomies", in patients with "idiopathic" or "persistent" floaters which had no or little objective correspondence (Roth et al. 2005; cf. Tausin 2005b). In clinical studies that evaluate the outcome of vitrectomies for floaters performed to relieve the patient's subjective strain, patients' satisfaction is strikingly high – around 90% (Schulz-Key et al. 2011; Weber-Varszegi et al. 2008). This figure must not be taken as a proof for the harmless floaters being vitreous opacities, though, for several reasons: in these studies, it is never entirely clear what kind of floaters these patients really had. Even if they are called "idiopathic", patients might not have seen the floater type at issue. Moreover, the patients' satisfaction is influenced by a number of factors such as visual improvement due to removing cataract and even subjective expectancy – the latter, together with the incomprehensible patients' strain as a motivation to get rid of floaters, tends to turn floaterectomy into a kind of psychotherapy (Tan et al. 2011; Tausin 2008). Also, there are many reports of patients that have experienced floaters after vitrectomy (Schulz-Key 2011; Degenerative Vitreous Community n/a). They are explained as remaining vitreous fibrils or newly developed floaters. Finally, if idiopathic floaters are no longer seen after FOV, there still might be other explanations for this. It is conceivable that the light is now channelled through the eye in a different (unstructured) way and, therefore, stimulates the retinal neurons differently, resulting in a vision with less or no floaters. Therefore, I suggest that the origin of floating spheres and strings should be looked for in the activity of visual neurology.

Conclusion

Present-day ophthalmology provides a frame to understand and describe the subjective visual spheres and strings known as harmless or idiopathic eye floaters. It is a historically grown melting pot in which floaters got associated with a number of eye disorders. A close observation of floaters reveals properties for which the disorder theory fails to provide a convincing explanation. Moreover, inconsistencies within this explanatory frame itself tell us to remain critical.

The spheres and strings are a subjective phenomenon. To study them means to be aware of that fact and to start from individual observation. We also have to keep in mind that perception is shaped not only by sensory data but also by our consciousness state, mental dispositions, motivations, cultural and social environments, etc. For example, it is my experience that size, luminosity and movement of floater spheres and strings alter according to different consciousness states. I think that understanding experiences like this is crucial in the search of a more reasonable understanding of floaters (Tausin 2009a). The subjective approach does not replace but complement and inform physiological research. For example, the observations presented in this article suggest considering the role of the visual nervous system in the process of seeing floaters.

References

Geller, Scott (n/a): "Is Laser Treatment an Option?". *Vitreousfloaters.com.* vitreousfloaters.com/faq.html (10.10.19)

Hirschberg, Julius (1899-1918): "Geschichte der Augenheilkunde". *Handbuch der gesamten Augenheilkunde 12-15*, ed. by E. Graefe and Th. Saemisch. Leipzig/Berlin: Springer

Johnson, James H. (n/a): "FAQ's for Young People with Eye Floaters". *Thefloaterdoctor.com.* thefloaterdoctor.com/young-floater-faqs/ (10.10.19)

Narasimhan, Arunn et al. (2015): "Convection-Enhanced Intravitreous Drug Delivery in Human Eye". *Journal of Heat Transfer 137*, no. 12

Narasimhan, Arunn et al. (2013): "Effect of choroidal blood perfusion and natural convection in vitreoushmor during transpupillary thermotherapy (TTT)". *International Journal for Numerical Methods in Biomedical Engineering 29*, no. 4

Plange, Hubertus (1990): "Muscae volitantes – von frühen Beobachtungen zu Purkinjes Erklärung". *Gesnerus 47:* 31-44

Roth, M. et al. (2005): "Pars-plana-Vitrektomie bei idiopathischen Glaskörpertrübungen". *Klinische Monatsblätter der Augenheilkunde 222*: 728-732

Sendrowski, David P.; Bronstein, Mark A. (2010): "Current treatment for vitreous floaters". *Optometry 81*: 157-161

Schulz-Key, Steffen et al. (2011): "Longterm follow-up of pars plana vitrectomy for vitreous floaters: complications, outcomes and patient satisfaction". *Acta Ophthalmologica 89*: 159-165

Tan, H. Stevie et al. (2011): "Safety of vitrectomy for floaters". *American Journal of Ophthalmology 151*, no. 6: 995-98

Tausin, Floco (2018): "Mouches volantes im antiken Griechenland. Teil 2: Magie, Mysterien, Fliegensehen und Philosophie". *Virtuelles Magazin 2000 82.* vm2000.net/8512/ (11.9.22)

Tausin, Floco (2010a): "Aus der Wissenschaft. Von aufsteigenden und absteigenden Mücken". *Ganzheitlich Sehen 1/10.* mouches-volantes.com/news/newsfebruar2010.htm#2 (11.9.22)

Tausin, Floco (2010b): "Eye Floaters. Floating spheres and strings in a seer's view". *Holistic Vision 2*. eye-floaters.info/news/news-june2010.htm#1 (11.9.22)

Tausin, Floco (2009a): *Mouches Volantes. Eye Floaters as Shining Structure of Consciousness*. Bern: Leuchtstruktur Verlag

Tausin, Floco (2009b): "Aus der Wissenschaft: Mouches volantes nicht im Glaskörper?" *Ganzheitlich Sehen 4/09*. mouches-volantes.com/news/newsdezember2009.htm#2 (11.9.22)

Tausin, Floco (2009c): "Mouches volantes – Glaskörpertrübung oder Nervensystem?" *Extremnews.com*, 22.12.09. extremnews.com/berichte/gesundheit/e01c12cc1d3c89f (11.9.22)

Tausin, Floco (2008): "Neues aus der Wissenschaft: 'Floaterektomie' als Psychotherapie?" *Ganzheitlich Sehen 3/08*. mouches-volantes.com/news/newsoktober2008.htm#4 (11.9.22)

Tausin, Floco (2005a): "Neues aus der Augenheilkunde: Nicht repräsentative Umfrage unter Augenärzten zum Thema 'Mouches volantes'". *Ganzheitlich Sehen*. mouches-volantes.com/news/newsaugust2005.htm (11.9.22)

Tausin, Floco (2005b): "Neues aus der Augenheilkunde: Klinische Studie über die Pars-plana-Vitrektomie bei Glaskörpertrübungen". *Ganzheitlich Sehen*. mouches-volantes.com/news/newsnovember2005.htm (11.9.22)

Weber-Varszegi, V. et al. (2008): "'Floaterektomie' – Pars-Plana-Vitrektomie wegen Glaskörpertrübungen". *Klinisches Monatsblatt Augenheilkunde 225*: 366-369

Links

Link[1]: *Sensitiveskinmagazine.com* (August 2011). sensitiveskinmagazine.com/in-depth-observations-on-eye-floaters-a-challenge-to-ophthalmology/ (11.9.22)

Link[2]: eyedoctorophthalmologistnyc.com/wp-content/uploads/2016/10/Eye-Floaters-Spots-treatment-nyc.jpg (11.9.22)

Link[3]: danielng.com.au/fiwee/?p=279 (15.6.11)

Link[4]: vitreousfloatersolutions.com/floatersyoung.html (11.6.11).

- "Floaters only vitrectomy". *Degenerative Vitreous.* tapatalk.com/groups/floatertalk/floaters-only-vitrectomy-f2/#.Tfh-e0djmy4 (11.9.22)

3
Do eye floaters arise from the visual nervous system?

First published:
Tausin, Floco (2011): "Vitreous opacity vs. nervous system – Do eye floaters arise from the visual nervous system?" Source: Link[1].

In ophthalmology, eye floaters are commonly considered to be a non-pathological age-related cloudiness of the vitreous body (Sendrowski 2010). According to this, vitreous structures that are clumped together cast shadows on the retina and become visible as mobile and transparent dots and strands in our field of vision.

In my opinion, this ophthalmological description of floaters as a "disorder" or "vitreous opacity" is a myth, based on too much theorizing and only superficial observation of the phenomenon. I suggest that floaters reflect a dualistic-polar organizing principle, which has, to some individuals, cultural or spiritual significance, but which also resembles the properties of receptive fields, an important aspect of the visual nervous system. To illustrate this, I firstly present important distinctive properties of floaters that are revealed through close observation, and then look for structural similarities in the neurology of vision. As an underlying theory, I assume that any phenomenal order in the perceptual experience corresponds with dynamic neurological organizing processes in the brain. This idea was originally developed as "isomorphism" by Gestalt psychologists (Köhler 1938; cf. Lehar 2003) and is – with regard to entoptic phenomena (cf. Trick 2007) – further reinforced by recent physiological research of entoptics, suggesting that these phenomena reflect the spatial organization of the neuronal structures of retina and cortex (Kent 2010; Bressloff et al. 2002; Cowan/Ermentrout 1979).

Floaters as receptive fields

In-depth observations of floaters reveal distinctive structures that are not considered and explained by ophthalmology (cf. Tausin 2011). Floater spheres are circular and concentric. They contain, clearly distinguishably, a core and a surround, viz. they are polar. The polarity is joined by a dualism, for there are two types of dots: those with a bright surround and a dark core, and those with a dark surround and a bright core. So we can speak of a dualistic-polar principle in floaters.

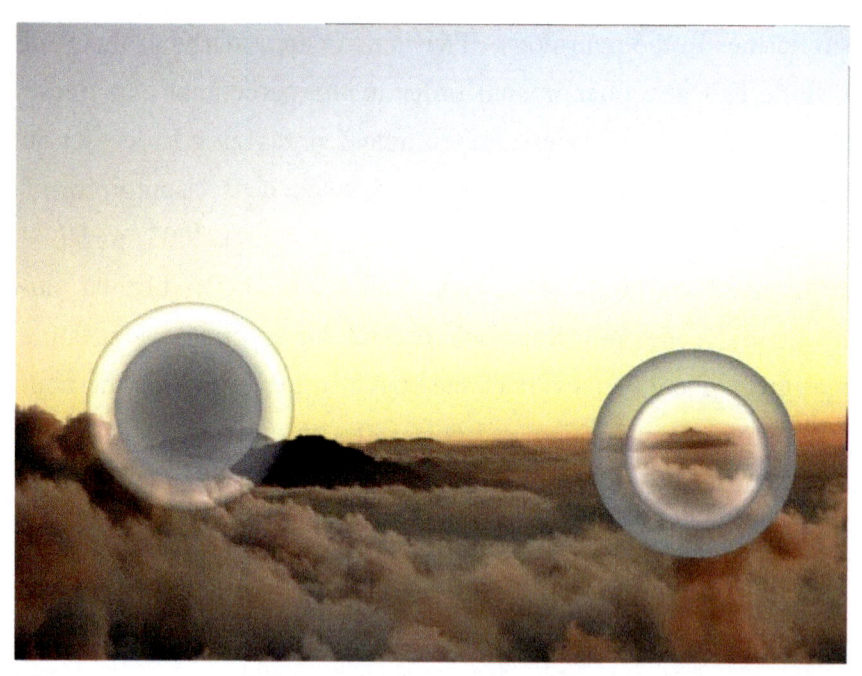

The two contrasting types of floater spheres. Source: Floco Tausin.

Morphologically, this principle is reflected in the visual nervous system. Nerve cells, or neurons, of the retina, the visual pathway and the visual cortices in the brain are also organized according to a dualistic-polar principle: the so-called receptive field (Freenlee/Tse 2008; Gareis/Lang 2007; Park 2007; Schiefer 2007; Witkovsky 2007; Goebel et al. 2004; Quillen/Barber 2002; Flores-Herr 2001; Greenstein/Greenstein 2000; cf. Franze 2007). To understand what receptive fields are, let's look at the way of the light in the visual pathway: light stimuli are first received by the light-sensitive receptors (retinal cones and rods) and forwarded through different layers of neurons. Cones and rods forward the stimuli to bipolar cells. The latter transmit the information to ganglion cells.

And from there, the impulses are forwarded through the neurites to the different neurons in the visual cortices in the brain.

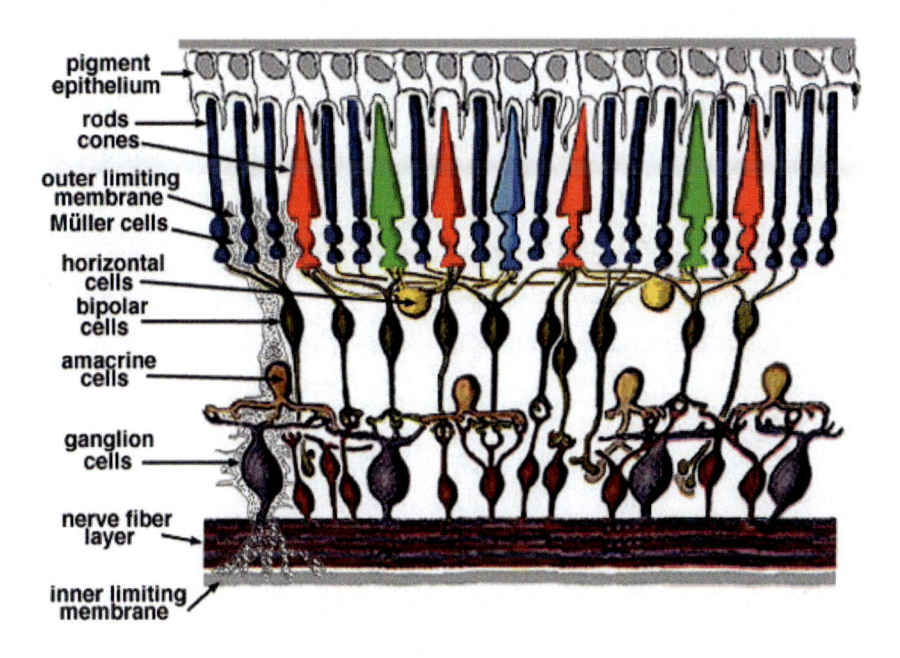

Simple diagram of the organization of the retina. Source: Link[2].

Bipolar, ganglion and the cortical neurons receive their light stimuli from their receptive field, a defined area in the visual field. For example, a bipolar cell answers to stimuli from cones and rods that belong to its receptive field. In turn, it forwards the stimulus to the ganglion cell to which receptive field it belongs. These receptive fields are circular concentric fields that are characterized by a centre and a surround. Therefore, the full technical term is "centre-surround antagonistic receptive field" (CSARF). There are two types of neurons that can be distinguished according to the function of their receptive fields: those that respond to light on their centre (on-centre) and those that respond to the illumination of their surround (on-periphery or off-centre). Stimulating photoreceptors in the centre of a receptive field of an on-centre bipolar cell excites the membrane of that bipolar cell (depolarization). The cell transmits this stimulus to the appropriate on-ganglion cell which likewise increases the discharge rate (action potentials per unit time). The same on-bipolar cell is inhibited (hyperpolarization) if its surround is illuminated, i.e. its discharge rate decreases. The off-centre bipolar cell behaves contrary: light on the centre decreases the discharge rate; light on the surround increases it.

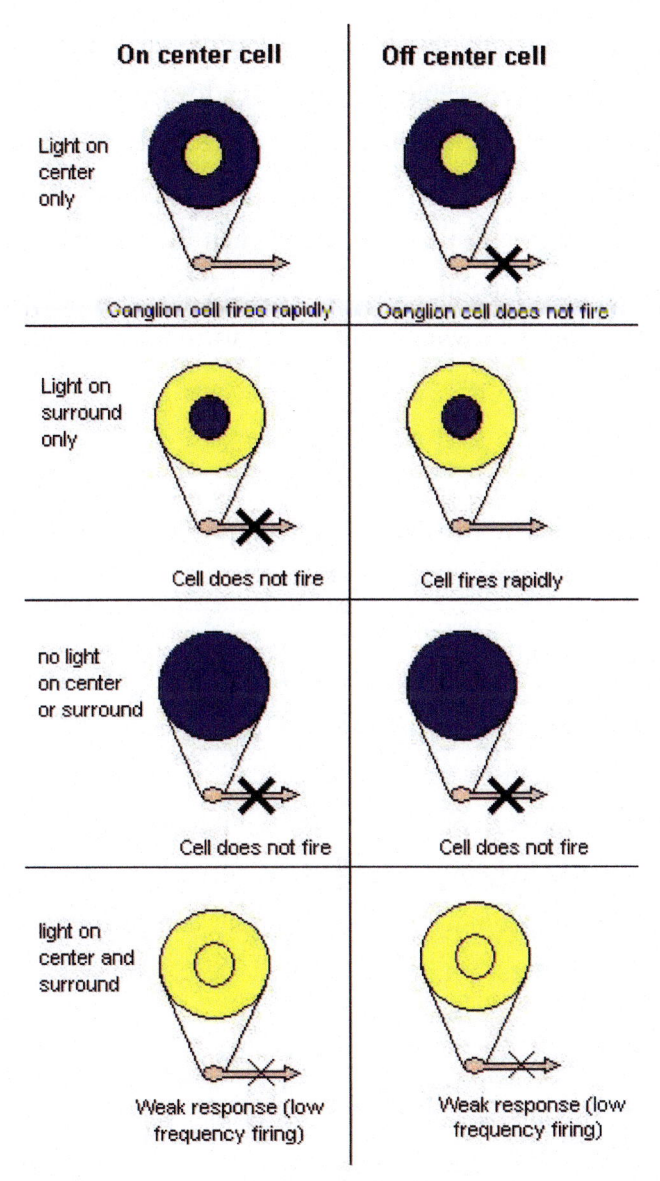

On centre and off centre retinal ganglion cells respond oppositely to light in the centre and surround of their receptive fields. A strong response means high frequency firing, a weak response is firing at a low frequency, and no response means no action potential is fired. Source: Link[3].

Both bipolar cells and ganglion cells receive their inputs not only from light sensitive receptors (vertical pathway) but also laterally from amacrine and horizontal cells (horizontal pathway). These forward the signals in the surround of a receptive field and cause the opposite reaction of each neuron when the surround is stimulated. Thus, amacrine and horizontal cells are part of the centre-surround antagonism which contributes to focused and distinctive vision.

From numerous neuronal responses to single scattered floaters: The consciousness principle

Both the receptive fields and the floater spheres are organized by the same dualistic-polar principle. This indicates the possibility that idiopathic floaters are not a "disorder" in the vitreous body, as advocated by modern ophthalmology, but an effect of the nervous system's visual light processing. The question is: how potent is that model in explaining further important and distinctive characteristics of floaters, as observed and described by the author (Tausin 2011)?

The most obvious question is how it comes that we actually see receptive fields. To answer that, let's have a look at the studies of mathematicians Bressloff et al. 2002 and Cowan/Ermentrout 1979 (cf. Meyers-Riggs 2011). They showed that entoptic patterns like phosphenes or form constants (Klüver 1966) arise from neuronal cortical structures. The cortical hypercolums – cells in the first layer of the visual cortex (V1) that respond to light input shaped as lines – are linked together in a manner that creates noise patterns of certain types. On the basis of the biological evidence that straight lines in the V1 are represented as curved lines on the retina, the researchers develop a mathematical model. Applied to the types of visual cortex noise, this model produces neuropsychologist Heinrich Klüver's types of form constants (a special kind of entoptic phenomena), which he described when experimenting with the psychedelic alkaloid mescaline (Klüver 1966).

These studies show that entoptic phenomena have a neuronal correlate. However, they do not address what I think is the main question: how and where exactly is the light that is received by the retina turned into visual consciousness? This is debated in today's (neuro-) ophthalmology (Goebel et al. 2004), as the neuronal correlate of consciousness is still a mystery to neurologists in general (Crick/Koch 1999). Fact is that visual experiences feed from external stimuli which are, however, neurally processed – they are constructions of the nervous system (cf. Lehar 2003). The cited studies seem to suggest that visual awareness (of entoptic phenomena) takes place only in the retina which is equated with the visual field. Many cognitive scientists, on the other hand, think that there are specific neurons in the cortex – in that case the visual cortex – that represent the neuronal correlate of consciousness (Goebel et al. 2004; Crick/Koch 1999). Contrary to this, I assume that visual awareness can take place in all of the neuronal layers of the visual pathway, from the retina to the higher layers of the visual cortex. I refer to the finding that simple visual forms correspond to earlier processing stages (retina, lower cortical layers) while more complex forms are extensively processed in higher layers of the optic centre (cf. Kent 2010; Goebel et al. 2004; Greenstein/Greenstein 2000). Therefore, I suggest that the visual experience of one and the same set of stimuli differs in terms of visual complexity and integration, depending on the level of neuronal processing on which visual awareness is aroused. Floaters, then, may be understood as the subjective visual realization of neuronal stimuli on an early (e.g. retinal, bipolar layer) stage of processing. The stimuli, canalized through receptive fields, are not yet processed to complex images, but transmit relatively simple and isolated properties such as shape and colour contrasts – the properties of receptive fields.

The question, then, is: What is this principle that decides on what level visual awareness gets aroused? Or, to put it another way, what is this principle that decides whether a nerve impulse comes to awareness as an isolated receptive field or floater, or whether we perceive it integrated and interpreted as a part of the image we call "the objective world"? For lack of a better term, I call it the "principle of consciousness". This consciousness principle might resolve the next question: if there is an abundance of receptive fields in the visual nervous system, why are we aware of just a few projected receptive fields in our visual field – just a few scattered floaters, respectively? I propose the following: on the one hand, this abundance can actually be seen as entoptic phenomena in certain circumstances – e.g. by squinting at the sun that reveals a whole "ocean of spheres" (Tausin 2010). On the other hand, the fact that floaters are indeed experienced as specific and persistent structure indicates that the consciousness principle brings a certain pattern of stimuli to visual awareness on an early level of neuronal processing. Referring to psychological or anthropological studies on entoptic phenomena and psychedelic drugs (e.g. Reichel-Dolmatoff 1978; Klüver 1966), I suggest that the consciousness principle does this according to the current state of consciousness of a person. According to this line of thinking, one might say that what we see in floaters is the neuronal correlate of our current state of consciousness. This is where the observation of floaters may have a spiritual significance to some individuals, if it is put into practice as a meditative investigation of one's own consciousness.

Movement

Another question concerns the obvious movement of floaters: If floaters are the visual expression of immobile receptive fields in the retina, in the visual pathway and the cortices – how can we understand their motion in our visual field, often even influenced by our own eye movements?

Here too, the consciousness principle provides a possible solution, along with the psychological concept of "apparent motion/movement". The latter designates moving impressions that do not arise from moving environmental stimuli, but from stationary stimuli, which are shown in sequence. As it is the case with cinematic images which are projected to the screen in rapid sequence and, thus, allowing our brain to experience a moved picture, our experience of moving floaters might be the result of successive stimulation of different, but self-similar retinal and cortical regions. In our theory, these effects may, however, not be caused by external stimuli alone, but by the consciousness principle. One objection to this might be that we obviously move our floaters by eye movements. My answer is that our physical movements cannot be separated from the consciousness principle: our physical activity is a result of our state of consciousness; conversely, physical and mental movements such as eye movements, concentration, emotions, etc. stimulate our nervous system, alter consciousness and, in that way, may cause perception of movement, or apparent motion respectively. There is even evidence suggesting the close connection between the activation of the muscles around the eyes and the perception of entoptic phenomena: rapid pulsation of eye muscles may be related to inhibiting or exciting the cortical columns that control optic muscles and may produce phosphenes (Kent 2010).

If correct, this means that we do not move our floaters with our eyes, but our eyes are moving in accordance with the dynamic, visually perceivable expression of our consciousness. It means that we are causing our floaters to flow or to stop by our psychophysical movements, or, to put it another way, by our consciousness.

Floater strings and receptive fields

Let's continue with another important observation: obviously, our floaters not only consist of spheres but also of strings. This might be the subjective visual expression of the fact that in certain cortical areas, the receptive fields of neurons are not circular and concentric, but elongated. They are strips of different spatial orientation. This means that neurons with elongated receptive fields strongly react to linear light stimuli like lines, columns, strips, etc. In addition, they are characterized by "orientation selectivity", i.e. they are pitched to particular angles and orientations of these light lines. In ophthalmology, it is not yet fully understood how the output of neurons with centre-surround receptive fields is translated into the orientation selectivity of the cortical neurons. A widely acknowledged hypothesis is that the elongated receptive fields in the cortex are, in fact, overlapping inputs of cells located in the lateral geniculate body. Those cells have, like bipolar and ganglion cells, circular receptive fields and end in the same receptive field of a cortical neuron (Goebel et al. 2004).

FIGURE 35.4 The mechanism by which the output of LGN cells with center-surround receptive fields is transformed into the elongated receptive fields of simple cortical cells is unknown. One hypothesis is that the simple cortical cell's receptive field is generated by the converging input of three or more ON-center LGN cells whose centers define its location and orientation. (Adapted from Kandel et al., 1995, p. 435).

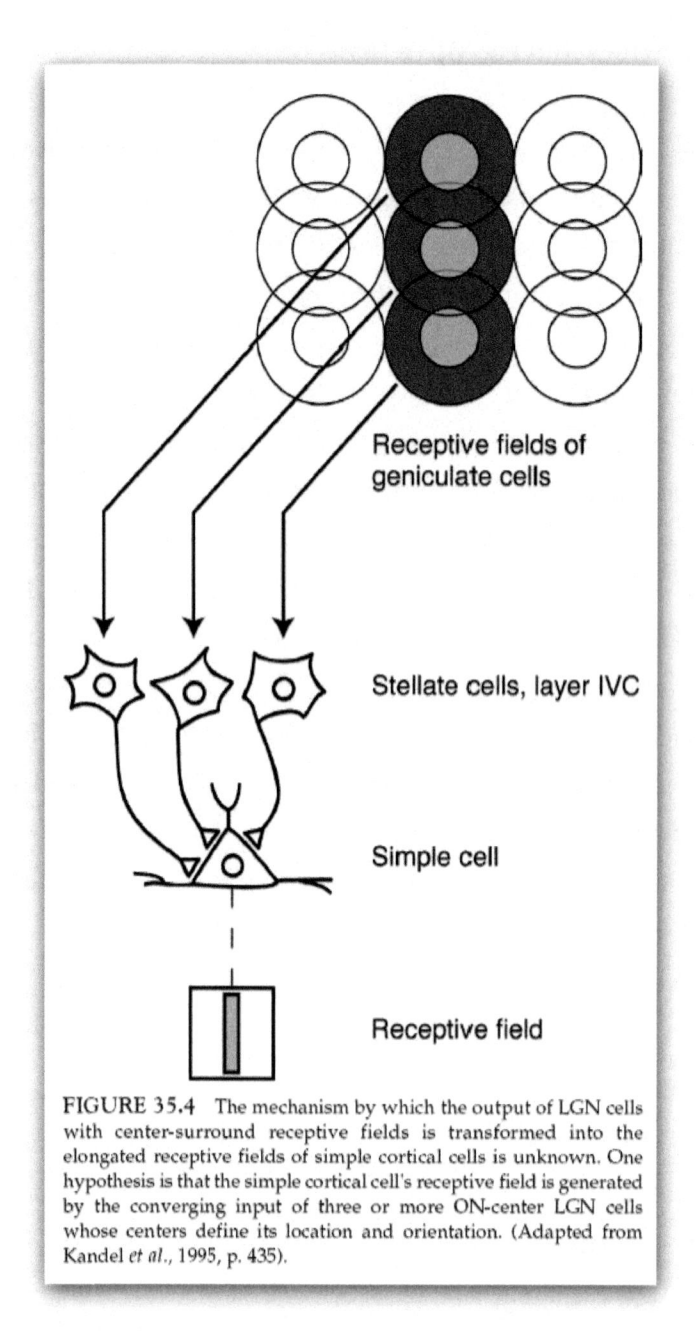

From floater spheres to floater strings? Source: Goebel et al. 2004.

Understanding floater strings as several spheres strung together not only corresponds to the subjective observation of floaters (although sometimes there are strings that seem to be empty); it also fits the fact that more complex forms – like floater strings filled with spheres – are represented by neurons in the higher visual centres of the brain (cf. Greenstein/Greenstein 2000; Goebel et al. 2004).

Explaining different light and size states in floaters neurologically

Another important, though not common, observation is that floater spheres and strings show different states over time: one and the same sphere can appear as big and rather hazy or as small and clearly outlined. The transition from one state to another is fluent and proceeds in different time duration. In general, it seems that most floaters are initially relaxed, viz. bigger, closer and more transparent; with increasing time of observation, they change into the concentrated state. In addition, the spheres and strings increase in brilliance the more concentrated they are (Tausin 2011).

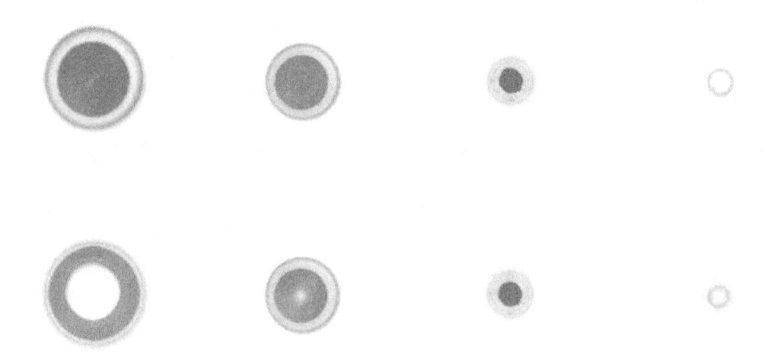

The two kinds of floater spheres in transition from a relaxed (left) to a concentrated (right) state. Source: Floco Tausin.

One possibility to explain this observation neurologically is to relate the floater size to the successive stimulation of different retinal and cortical regions. While in case of the observation of lateral or horizontal movements of floaters (see above), these regions are successively stimulated laterally, here they are stimulated vertically. In other words, the transition from one floater state to another corresponds to the transition of visual awareness from one neuronal layer to another. The simple and abstract information of every neuronal layer differs not in shape, but in size.

Let's turn to the changing luminosity in floaters. How come that we perceive light in floaters at all? An answer is provided by Hungarian bioengineer István Bókkon who, referring to the phenomenon of bioluminescence, suggests that neurons emit light which we can perceive. He shows that nerve cells can transform electrical signals through processes of bioluminescence into ultraweak light. This light, or the emitted biophotons respectively, not only serves the intra- and intercellular communication, but can be perceived by us as entoptic phenomenon, e.g. as phosphenes (Bókkon 2009, 2008). It is thus conceivable that the light in floaters arises from varying electrical/biophotonic discharge of neurons. The theory of awareness on different neuronal layers, together with the notion of light emission of discharging neurons, is sufficient to explain the relationship of size and luminosity observed in floaters: when we are in concentrated states of consciousness, visual awareness takes place in "lower" neuronal layers (I suggest: closer to the retina) with cells firing faster; being in more relaxed states of consciousness corresponds to visual awareness on "higher" layers with neurons less excited. This whole process is controlled by the consciousness principle, but also influenced by exterior stimuli.

Conclusion

In this article, I have proposed a neurological explanation of eye floaters. A particular structure of neuronal processing seems to correspond to the structure of floater spheres and strings: the receptive field. Starting from receptive fields, I tried to understand some of the more important observations of floaters in terms of neuronal processing, assuming a "consciousness principle" that decides on what stage of processing visual awareness is experienced.

This work cannot prove the claims it has made. Rather, the text is intended to give new impetus to the further exploration of so-called floaters, starting from subjective observation. Especially the inclusion of the subject allows for a variety of different interpretations and explanations, not only ophthalmological or neurological, but also psychological, historical, anthropological and spiritual – a step towards a comprehensive science, which can complement isolated academic accounts on eye floaters and other entoptic phenomena.

References

Bókkon, István (2008): "Phosphene phenomenon: A new concept". *BioSystems 92*: 168-174

Bókkon István (2009): "Visual perception and imagery: A new molecular hypothesis". *BioSystems 96*: 178-184.
5mp.cu/fajlok/bokkon-brain-imagery/visual_perception_and_imagery,_a_new_molecular_hypothesis_bokkon_2009_www.5mp.eu_.pdf (11.9.22)

Bressloff, P. C. et al. (2002): "What Geometric Visual Hallucinations Tell Us about the Visual Cortex". *Neural Computation 14*: 473-491

Cowan, J. D.; Ermentrout, G. B. (1979): "A Mathematical Theory of Visual Hallucination Patterns". *Biol. Cybernetics 34*: 137-150.
math.pitt.edu/~bard/pubs/Ermentrout-Cowan79b.pdf (10.10.19)

Crick, Christof; Koch, Francis (1999): "Consciousness, Neurobiology of". *The MIT Encyclopedia of Cognitive Sciences,* ed. by Robert A. Wilson and Frank C. Keil. Cambridge/MA: The MIT Press: 193-194.

Flores-Herr, Nicolas (2001): *Das hemmende Umfeld von Ganglienzellen in der Netzhaut des Auges* (Dissertation im Fachbereich Physik, Johann-Wolfgang-Goethe-Universität, Frankfurt a.M.). d-nb.info/963919318/34 (11.9.22)

Franze, Kristian (2007): "Lichtleiter in der Netzhaut". *Spektrum der Wissenschaft 10:* 16-19

Greenlee, Mark W.; Tse, Peter U. (2008): "Functional Neuroanatomy of the Human Visual System: A Review of Functional MRI Studies". *Pediatric Ophthalmology, Neuro-Ophthalmology, Genetics (Essentials in Ophthalmology)*, ed. by B. Lorenz and F.-X. Bourrat. Berlin/Heidelberg: Springer: 119-138

Greenstein, Ben; Greenstein, Adam (2000): Color *Atlas of Neuroscience. Neuroanatomy and Neurophysiology*. Stuttgart/NY: Thieme

Gareis, Oskar; Lang, Gerhard K. (2007): "Visual Pathway". *Ophthalmology. A Pocket Textbook Atlas,* ed. by Gerhard K. Lang. Stuttgart/NY: Thieme: 401-414

Goebel, Rainer et al. (2004): "Visual System". The Human Nervous System (2nd ed.), ed. by Geroge Paxinos et al. San Diego: *Academic Press*: 1280-1305

Kentridge, Robert; Heywood, Charles; Davidoff, Jules (2003): "Color Perception". *Handbook of Brain Theory and Neural Networks*, ed. by Michael A. Arbib. Cambridge/London: MIT Press

Klüver, Heinrich (1966): *Mescal and the Mechanisms of Hallucination*. Chicago: University of Chicago Press

Köhler, Wolfgang (1938): *The Place of Value in a World of Facts*. Liveright Publishing Corporation.

Lehar, Steven (2003): "Gestalt Isomorphism and the Primacy of Subjective Conscious Experience: A Gestalt Bubble Model". *Behavioral and Brain Sciences 26*: 375-444. dartmouth.edu/~peter/pdf/15.pdf (10.10.19)

Meyers-Riggs, Bill (2011). "Form Constants and the Visual Cortex". *Countyourculture.com*. countyourculture.com/2011/03/13/form-constants-visual-cortex/ (10.10.19)

Park, Susanna S. (2007): "The Anatomy and Cell Biology of the Retina". *Duane's Ophthalmology*, ed. by William Tasman and Edward A. Jaeger. Philadelphia: Lippincott Williams & Wilkins [electronic edition]

Plange, Hubertus (1990): "Muscae volitantes – von frühen Beobachtungen zu Purkinjes Erklärung". *Gesnerus 47*: 31-44

Quillen, David A.; Barber, Alistair, J. (2002): "Anatomy and Physiology of the Retina". Clinical Retina, ed. by David A. Quillen and Barbara A. Blodi. *American Medical Association (AMA)*

Reichel-Dolmatoff, Gerardo (1978): *Beyond the Milky Way. Hallucinatory Imagery of the Tukano Indians*. Los Angeles: University of California

Roth, M.; Trittibach, P.; Koerner, F; Sarra, G. (2005): "Pars-plana-Vitrektomie bei idiopathischen Glaskörpertrübungen". *Klinische Monatsblätter der Augenheilkunde 222*: 728-732

Schiefer, U; Hart, W. (2007): "Functional Anatomy of the Human Visual Pathway". *Clinical Neuro-Ophthalmology. A Practical Guide*, ed. by Ulrich Schiefer, Helmut Wilhelm and William Hart. Berlin/Heidelberg: Springer: 19-28

Sendrowski, David P.; Bronstein, Mark A. (2010): "Current treatment for vitreous floaters". *Optometry 81*: 157-161

Tausin, Floco (2011): "In-depth observations on eye floaters – A challenge to ophthalmology". *Sensitiveskinmagazine.com* (August 2011). sensitiveskinmagazine.com/in-depth-observations-on-eye-floaters-a-challenge-to-ophthalmology/ (11.9.22)

Tausin, Floco (2010): "Mouches volantes und Makulachagrin". *Ganzheitlich Sehen 4/10*. mouches-volantes.com/news/newsdezember2010.htm#2 (11.9.22)

Tausin, Floco (2009): *Mouches Volantes. Eye Floaters as Shining Structure of Consciousness*. Bern: Leuchtstruktur Verlag

Trick, Gary L.; Kronenberg, Alaina (2007): "Entoptic Imagery and Afterimages". *Duane's Ophthalmology*, ed. by William Tasman and Edward A. Jaeger. Philadelphia: Lippincott Williams & Wilkins [electronic edition]

Weber-Varszegi, V.; Senn, P.; Becht, V. N.; Schmid, M. K. (2008): "'Floaterektomie' – Pars-Plana-Vitrektomie wegen Glaskörpertrübungen". *Klinisches Monatsblatt Augenheilkunde 225*: 366-369

Werblin, Frank; Roska, Botond (2008): "Wie das Auge die Welt verfilmt". *Spektrum der Wissenschaft 5*: 41-47

Witkovsky, Paul (2007): "Functional Anatomy of the Retina". *Duane's Ophthalmology*, ed. by William Tasman and Edward A. Jaeger. Philadelphia: Lippincott Williams & Wilkins [electronic edition]

Links

Link[1]: *Ovi Magazine*, 31.10.11. ovimagazine.com/art/7852 (11.9.22)

Link[2]: selflearningvisionsystem.blogspot.com/2009/07/httpwebvision.html (11.9.22)

Link[3]: psychology.wikia.org/wiki/Visual_receptive_fields (11.9.22).

4
The Spiritual Dimension of the Migraine Aura

First published:
Tausin, Floco (2010): "Migraine Aura: Suggestions for Spiritual Approaches to Migraine Headaches". Source: Link[1].

In spring 2007, I received an email from Klaus Podoll, MD, deputy of the Clinic for Psychiatry and Psychotherapy at the University Hospital in Aachen, Germany. He is editor of the Migraine Aura Foundation, dedicated to classifying and understanding migraine headaches and migraine auras in order to help patients, and to exploring human brain functioning in cognitive and psychological processes. Dr. Podoll read about my work on eye floaters and spirituality. He wanted to know if I knew about the phenomenon of migraine aura – the subjective visual phenomena preceding migraine headaches – and, if so, what my position about that phenomenon would be.

To me, this was a surprising and unusual inquiry, for my research methods are humanistic and spiritual rather than medical. However, it turned out that Dr. Podoll collects and presents alternative approaches for the Migraine Aura Foundation, including the areas of art and spirituality. He has pragmatic reasons for this, since such approaches can have positive results in the therapy of migraine patients. This may be viewed as an expression of the dialogues about the reintegration of religion into medicine, taking place since the 1990s.

In Western culture, religion and medicine have been closely interwoven for centuries. It was only with the rise of materialistic and empiricist worldviews in the 17th century that medicine shifted to focus solely on empirically verifiable processes, excluding 'supernatural' or spiritual effects on human health. In the last 30 years, however, it was shown in a number of studies that treatment of complaints and illnesses like diabetes, liver disorders, heart conditions, cancer, arthritis and chronic pains are facilitated if the patient is spiritually active. While the mechanisms for the physical effects of religion and spirituality have not been clarified yet, it is generally acknowledged that religions regulate the feelings of the people and therefore have an effect on the immune system and the psyche (Koenig 2003; Slager Johnson/Kushner 2001; Niv 2001; Parris/Smith 2003).

This article is an answer to Dr. Podoll's inquiry and a contribution to the developments in medicine outlined above. It examines the migraine aura from a spiritual view, and explores migraine not only a physical but also as a spiritual condition which is accessible to conscious alterations.

Migraine headaches

Migraine headaches may be unilateral or bilateral, pulsating headaches frequently accompanied by an increased sensitivity to light and noise, by nausea and dizziness, sometimes even by abdominal cramps, numbness in various parts of the body and temporary paralysis. The duration of this condition ranges from several hours up to several days. There are different neurophysiological theories about the causes of migraine, focusing primarily on changes in the blood circulation of the brain or on neural excitation. Genetic factors may also contribute to the occurrence of migraines.

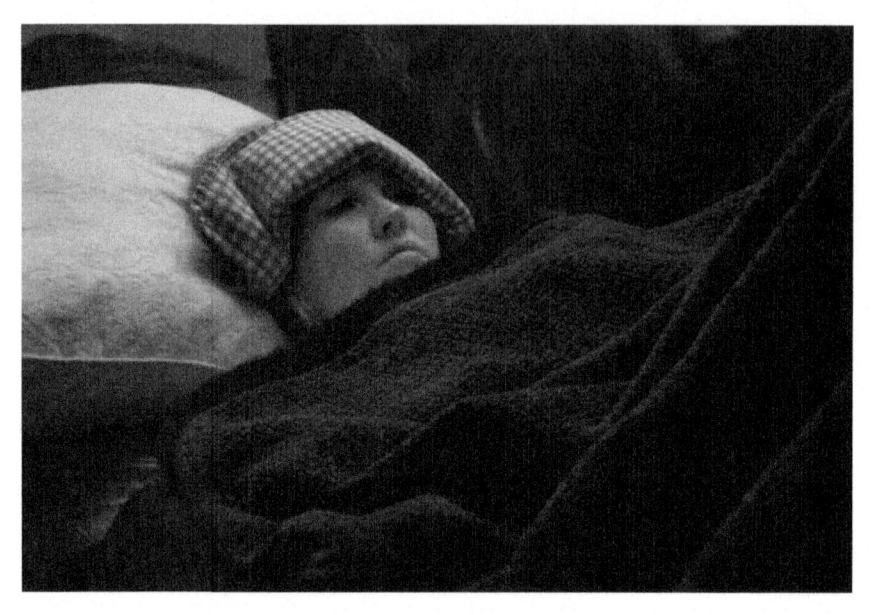

Suffering from migraine headache. Source: Link[2].

A great number of factors are known to trigger migraines, including stimulants like chocolate, coffee, red wine and salt food; hormonal changes in the body; emotional strains; climatic conditions; and others (Rowland/Frey 2005; Dalsgaard-Nielsen 1973). Approximately 12-14% of women and 8% of men are affected by migraine in the industrial nations of Western Europe and the USA, thus causing several billion dollars in costs every year for medical treatments and absenteeism from work (Reuter 2005).

I find it of note that authors like Stephen King and Steven Sills create protagonists who suffer from migraine to point to events lying ahead, or to start a process of reflection. Wassily Kandinsky, Yayoi Kusama, Lewis Carroll, Giorgio de Chirico, Sarah Raphael and other visual artists have let themselves be inspired to works of art by migraine experiences (cp. Dahlem and Podoll, 16.11.09).

Alternative treatments of migraine

The broad incidence of migraines is reflected in a wide array of treatments outside of conventional medicine. Some of these approaches stem from medieval or pre-Christian European medical systems; others derive from non-Western medicine. Some very old magical and alchemical practices and recipes have been recommended for treatment of migraine (Eggetsberger 1992; Retschlag 1934). Other therapies understand "illness as a way" (Dethlefsen and Dahlke 1997; Schwendener 2000) and try to find the spiritual causes of migraine. Yet other approaches focus primarily on the spiritual development of man, where the cure of diseases is "only" a welcome side effect. Western complementary and alternative medicine often isolates methodologies from such approaches from their cultural and religious roots for use against migraine. Therapies that report success in migraine treatment include acupuncture and acupressure, homoeopathy, meditation, Neuro-Linguistic Programming (NLP), sensory deprivation, shiatsu, yoga, autogenic training, as well as prayers and spirituality in general (Rowland and Frey 2005).

The visual migraine aura – an entoptic phenomenon

In these alternative approaches, the focus practically never lies on the migraine aura that precedes the migraine in a minority of persons affected (10-20 %). In ancient medicine the Greek term *aúra* described the pre-symptom of an epileptic seizure. In the case of migraine, it serves to describe subjective "imaginary" sensory perceptions, which precede the headaches for one hour at most. Although auras can affect all senses, they usually refer to the visual sense (Göbel, 16.11.09; Dahlem and Podoll, 16.11.09).

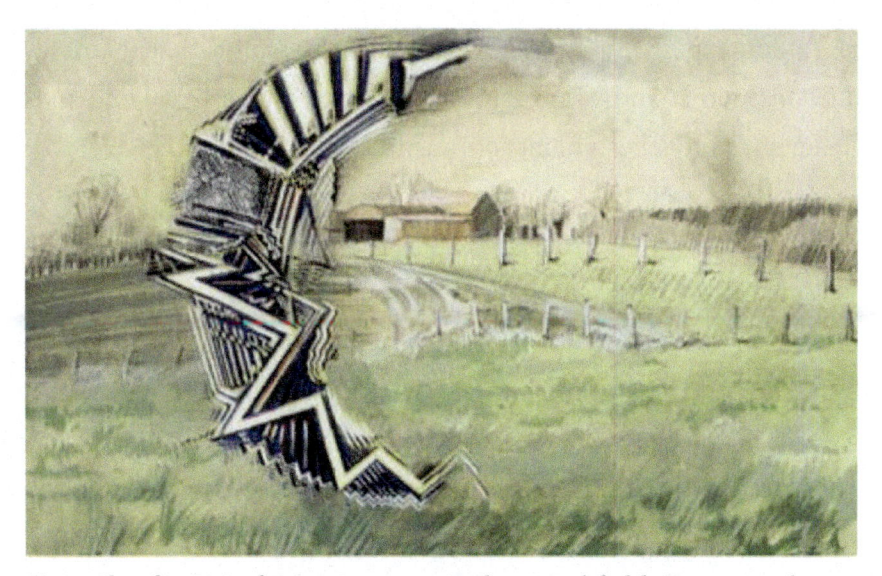

Example of a typical migraine aura in the visual field. Drawing of a patient. Source: Dodick 2009.

A visual aura may manifest in several different variations, being composed of typical and atypical visual phenomena. Atypical visual phenomena like small bright dots, white, coloured or dark spots, zigzags, lines, flashes of light, "foggy vision" and others, are most frequent (Queiroz et al. 1997). Typical visual phenomena include a flicker (scintillation) and the visual field defect (scotoma). Both can extend and move in the visual field.

All these appearances can be understood as 'entoptic phenomena', a medical term for a specific group of subjective visual phenomena, some of which we know from more common, everyday experiences reported by people who do not have migraines. Entoptic phenomena include 'form constants', moving geometric patterns; complementary coloured afterimages; tiny luminous spheres moving along rapidly in spiral tracks known as 'blue field entoptic phenomenon'; and transparent dots and strings called 'eye floaters' or mouches volantes (Tausin 2006b, 2006c).

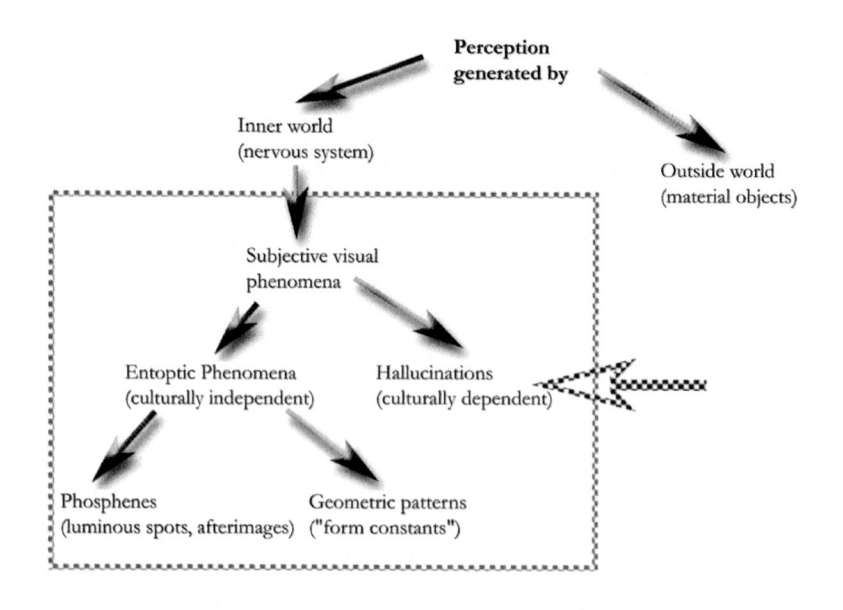

Kinds of subjective visual phenomena. Source: Floco Tausin.

Intensity increase and altered consciousness

The interpretation of migraine represented here takes the entoptic phenomena as a starting point. In many cultures practicing ritual forms of deep consciousness alteration, these phenomena are highly valued in their religion, art and society (Bednarik et al. 1990; Tausin 2006a, 2007a). Apart from ecstasy techniques practiced by shamans and seers, migraine can also be a trigger for entoptic perceptions. As early as the 1980s, the doctors J. Dexter and

A. Friedman noted similarities in the altered central nervous system of migraine patients and of shamans in states of trance (Dexter and Friedman 1984). And the ethnopharmacologist Christian Rätsch, in his *Encyclopedia of Psychoactive Plants*, draws attention to the perception changes in migraine and in ritual trance states induced by active agents of plants, in both cases triggered by the activation of certain neurotransmitters (Rätsch 2005).

All of this suggests that migraine sufferers experience a stimulation of the nervous system in the phase of the aura which I call an "intensity increase" or "heightened energy metabolism" (Tausin 2009a). According to medical reports, this energy surge frequently manifests before the appearance of the aura and engenders a good mood, effusive joy and openness, or intensive sadness, fear and depression in people affected. Bodily sensations like prickling, tingling and shivering, which are frequently experienced by migraine patients during the aura phase, are a further sign of increased energy.

In some religious traditions, such feelings normally appear at moments of intense emotions and are a sign for the openness towards the divine. This temporary increase in energy as well as the ability to deal with that energy is often interpreted as having a spiritual meaning, because it changes the consciousness and the perception of people. This was sought by ecstatics, mystics, shamans and visionaries of all times and cultures to facilitate contact with the divine (Tausin 2007b).

While shamans and ecstatics, however, are preparing themselves physically and spiritually over many years for such intensity increases and perception changes, migraine sufferers are thrown "into the cold water" without preparation or spiritual support. I suggest that some appear able to process this increase in energy, as seen in the fact that in these cases there is no headache following the visual auras (e.g. Waterwolf, 16.11.09). Most migraine sufferers, however, lack the physical and spiritual prerequisites to handle that situation: the increased energy can't flow freely and evenly in the body – which expresses itself as the typical migraine symptoms of headaches, nausea and oversensitivity.

Entoptic spirituality to counteract migraines

From the point of view of the ecstatics, migraine sufferers are generally more open to altered states of consciousness because they experience frequent energy increases – even if these are uninvited and uncontrolled. This means that if migraine patients are willing to work ecstatically, they have a chance not only to control this increased energy, and thus to get rid of the unwanted migraine symptoms, but also to develop their own consciousness as well.

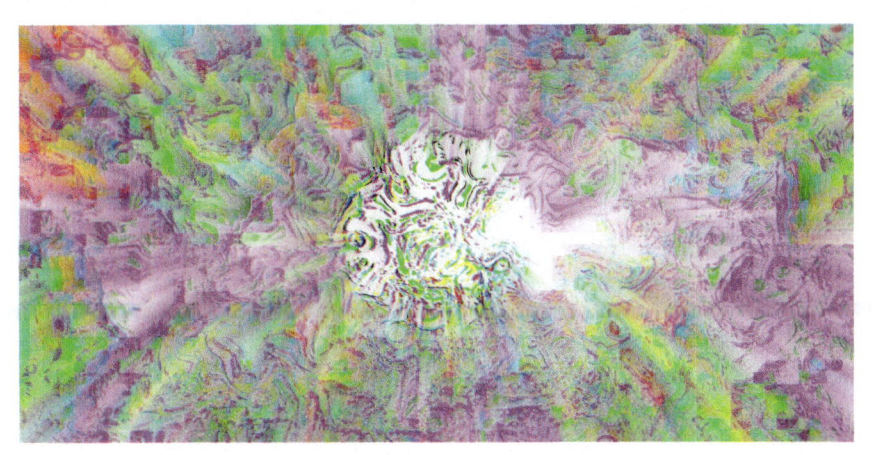

Migraine aura. By Joana Roja. Source: Link[3].

We can find the inspirations for this ecstatic-energetic work in religions and spiritual teachings which include entoptic phenomena. According to my previous enquiries, aspects of an "entoptic spirituality" can be found in practices and beliefs of shamanistic societies, in the mystical and visionary traditions of Hinduism, Buddhism, Christianity and Islam, as well as in modern teachings like the esoteric aura, the theory of Orgone by Wilhelm Reich, or the mystic teaching of the seer Nestor living in the Swiss Emmental (Tausin 2006a, 2006b, 2009a).

The phenomena of entopic spirituality provide at least three helpful suggestions for migraine treatment. First, they reframe entoptic phenomena in personal and cosmic contexts and thus convert them into positive and meaningful experiences. In this way, they provide intellectual frameworks for interpreting migraine auras, and therefore migraines in general, within the religious or spiritual traditions of migraine sufferers. So far, there is no empirical data available to make statements about the efficacy of such specific intellectual frameworks in migraine patients. But the case of U.S. artist Robert Bursik shows the healing power of spiritual explanations in migraine aura patients in general: Bursik connected these perceptions with statements from different religions and assigned the cause to spirit. His headaches disappeared after he had accepted the auras, which at first had generated fears (Bursik, 16.11.09).

Second, entoptic spirituality requires a change in daily behaviour. It provides the concrete physical and spiritual practices, suitable to prepare for this recurring situation of increased energy. If integrated into one's daily schedule and exercised for some time, such practices help remove subtle energy blocks, which, within understandings of biological energy fields, may cause pains and other symptoms (Benor 2001; Brennan 1988).

Practices of mystics and ecstatics that may be relevant to treating migraines may include many health-promoting practices:

- healthy, balanced vegetarian or vegan food;
- regular walks in fresh air as well as physical exercises aimed at the flexibility and sensitivity of the body, e.g. dance, yoga, tai chi etc.;
- breathing exercises;
- concentration, meditation and relaxation exercises.

Reports from complementary and alternative medicine confirm that these exercises and practices have been helpful in treatment of migraines (Rowland/Frey 2005). In that way, migraine pains motivate spiritual activity, which again shows the close connectedness of medicine and religion. For many religious or spiritual traditions or philosophies are results of the aspiration to alleviate or transcend pains. That's how the philosopher Marcel Proust's statement on illness helps us understand why religious traditions are often followed with much devotion and zeal when pains are present: "Illness is the doctor to whom we pay most heed; to kindness, to knowledge, we make promises only; to pain we obey."

Third, entoptic spirituality stresses the importance of experiencing and examining entoptic phenomena as consciously as possible, resulting in a kind of open eye meditation (Tausin 2009b). Similarly, migraine sufferers working ecstatically are encouraged to observe their auras very attentively. In this exercise, the two above mentioned aspects meet: the intellectual framework tells the aura observers that they experience something sacred during these moments; helps them to break free from their usual thinking, acting and perceiving for a period of time; and invites them to experience the world in a new way. This is something that ecstatics and shamans work for all their life. The physical exercises mentioned help to deal with the energy increase and thus to maintain a clear consciousness during these moments. I propose that, just as meditation on eye floaters relieves the anxieties that may be connected with them (Tausin 2009a), meditation on auras will result in overcoming the fears and anxieties accompanying this condition.

My suggestion is that the combination of these aspects of entoptic spirituality will help migraine sufferers to cope better with their migraine auras and migraine symptoms. There is no data as yet to support this suggestion. Again, Robert Bursik may be taken as a successful example who demonstrates at least some of the above mentioned aspects, including a redefining intellectual framework and close observation of the phenomena. Thanks to the spiritual interpretation and his patience, he has been able to enjoy the auras for three decades:

> "And if I let it, and take time, and watch it, it slows down, and I can enjoy the simple beauty of it for what it is."

References

Bednarik, Robert G.; Lewis-Williams, J. D.; Dowson, Thomas A. (1990): "On Neuropsychology and Shamanism in Rock Art". *Current Anthropology 31*, no. 1: 77-84

Benor, Daniel J. (2007): Healing Research: Volume I, Spiritual Healing: *Scientific Validation of a Healing Revolution*. Wholistic Healing Publications

Brennan, Barbara A. (1988): *Hands of Light: A Guide to Healing Through the Human Energy Field*, NY: Bantam

Bursik, Robert V. (2009): "Migraines: My story – my solution". *Migraine-aura.org*. migraine-aura.org/content/e27891/e27265/e42715/e42749/e46723/index_en.html (16.11.09)

Dahlem, Markus; Podoll, Klaus (2009): *Migraine Aura*. migraine-aura.org (11.9.22)

Dahlke, Rüdiger; Dethlefsen, Thorwald; Lemesurier, Peter (1997): *The Healing Power of Illness. The Meaning of Symptoms and How to Interpret Them* (German title: Krankheit als Weg, 1990). Element Books Ltd.

Dalsgaard-Nielsen, T. (1973): "The Nature of Migraine. Delivered in abbreviated form as a lecture at the Annual Meeting of the American Association for the Study of Headache in New York on 23rd June". *Headache. The Journal of Head and Face Pain 14*, no. 1: 13-25

Dexter, J.; Friedman, A. (1984): "The myth and magic of migraine therapy. A look into the shaman's bag". *Progress in Migraine Research 2*, ed. by F. Rose. London: 265-268

Duerden, Tim (2004): "An aura of confusion: 'seeing auras – vital energy or human physiology?' Part 1 of a three part series". *Complementary Therapies in Nursing & Midwifery 10*: 22-29

Eggetsberger, Gerhard H. (1992): *Hypnose. Die unheimliche Realität. Selbsthypnose, Fremdhypnose, Hypnose im Alltag.* Wien et al.

Göbel, Hartmut; Heinze, Axel; Heinze-Kuhn, Katja (2009): *Die Morgendämmerung der Migräne – die Auraphase*. migraeneliga-deutschland.de/die-auraphase.htm (16.11.09)

Ilacqua, G.E. (1994): "Migraine headaches. Coping efficacy of guided imagery training". *Headache 34:* 99-102

Koenig, Harold G. (2003): "Medicine". *Encyclopaedia of Science and Religion*, ed. by J. Wentzel Vrede van Huyssteen et al. New York: Macmillan Reference: 552-556

Monrad, Jorunn (200): Entoptic phenomena in contemporary art. (The original website *entopticart.com* has expired. It can be retrieved at: web.archive.org/web/20080605024658/http://www.entopticart.com/ (11.9.22))

Niv, David; Kreitler, Shulamith (2001): "Pain and Quality of Life". *Pain Practice 1*, no. 2: 150-161

Parris, Winston C. V.; Smith, Howard S. (2003): "Alternative Pain Medicine". *Pain Practice 3*, no. 2: 105-116

Queiroz, Luiz P. et al. (1997): "Characteristics of Migraine Visual Aura". *Headache 37*: 137-141

Rätsch, Christian (2005): *The Encyclopedia of Psychoactive Plants. Ethnopharmacology and Its Applications*. Park Street Press

Retschlag, Max (1934): *Die Alchimie und ihr grosses Meisterwerk der Stein der Weisen*. Leipzig: Richard Hummel Verlag

Reuter, Uew (2004): Pathomechanismen der Migräne (*Habilitationsschrift, eingereicht an Medizinischen Fakultät der Charité, Universitätsmedizin Berlin)*. edoc.hu-berlin.de/habilitationen/reuter-uwe-2004-06-21/HTML/chapter1.html (11.9.22)

Roach, Mary (1998): "Ancient Altered States". *Discover 19*, 6.

Rowland, Belinda; Frey, Rebecca J. (2009): "Migraine headache". *The Gale Encyclopaedia of alternative medicine (3rd ed.)*, ed. by Laurie J. Fundukian: 1497-1502

Slager Johnson, Susan; Kushner, Robert F. (2001): "Mind/Body Medicine: An Introduction for the Generalist Physician and Nutritionist". *Nutrition in Clinical Care 4*, no. 5: 256–264

Schwendener, Urs (2000): Anthroposophie. Die Geisteswissenschaft Rudolf Steiners. *Ein alphabetisches Nachschlagewerk in 14 Bänden*. Oberdorf

Steiger, Brad; Steiger, Sherry Hansen (2003): "Hallucinations". *The Gale Encyclopedia of the Unusual and Unexplained (Vol. 3)*, ed. by Brad Steiger. Detroit et al.: 143

Tausin, Floco (2009a): *Mouches Volantes. Eye Floaters as Shining Structure of Consciousness*. Bern: Leuchtstruktur Verlag

Tausin, Floco (2009b): "Open Eye Meditation. The visual way to the development of the inner sense". *International Journal of Healing and Caring 9*, no. 3. eye-floaters.info/articles-archive/floco_tausin__open_eye_meditation.pdf (11.9.22)

Tausin, Floco (2007a): "'Entoptic Art' – Entoptische Erscheinungen als Inspirationsquelle in der zeitgenössischen bildenden Kunst". *ExtremNews.com*, 29.1.07. extremnews.com/berichte/vermischtes/396b116f79905e4 (11.9.22)

Tausin, Floco (2007b): "Wenn sich die Haare sträuben. Das Prickeln auf der Haut als universelles spirituelles Phänomen". *Esotera 1*

Tausin, Floco (2006a): "Mouches volantes und Trance. Ein universelles Phänomen bei erweiterten Bewusstseinszuständen früher und heute". *Jenseits des Irdischen 3*

Tausin, Floco (2006b): "Mouches volantes. Bewegliche Kugeln und Fäden aus der Sicht eines Sehers". *Q'Phase. Realität ... Anders! 4*

Tausin, Floco (2006c): "Zwischen Innenwelt und Aussenwelt. Entoptische Phänomene und ihre Bedeutung für Bewusstseinsentwicklung und Spiritualität". *Schlangentanz 3*

Waterwolf. "Migraine Symptoms Without Headaches". *Essortment*. essortment.com/articles/migraine-symptoms-headaches_104450.htm (16.11.09)

Links

Link[1]: *International Journal of Healing and Caring 10*, no. 1. irp-cdn.multiscreensite.com/891f98f6/files/uploaded/Tausin-10-1.pdf (11.9.22)

Link[2]: farm3.static.flickr.com/2045/2450239227_ce9850c377.jpg?v=0 (11.9.22)

Link[3]: flickr.com/photos/cats_mom/2758240218/ (11.9.22)

- entopticart.com/ (2009)
- migraene.msd.de/wissen/defi/miga_1140.html (2009)
- dr-gumpert.de/html/migraene.html (11.9.22)
- wdr.de/themen/gesundheit/krankheit/migraene/050901.jhtml (2009)

- medizin.uni-koeln.de/stan/Schmerzmanual/KS/ddmispa.html (2009)
- migraeneliga-deutschland.de/die-auraphase.htm (2009)
- discover.com/issues/jun-98/features/ancientalteredst1456/ (21.6.06)
- migraine-aura.org (11.9.22)
- mail-archive.com/assam@pikespeak.uccs.edu/msg04629.html (11.9.22)

The author

Floco Tausin
floco.tausin@eye-floaters.info

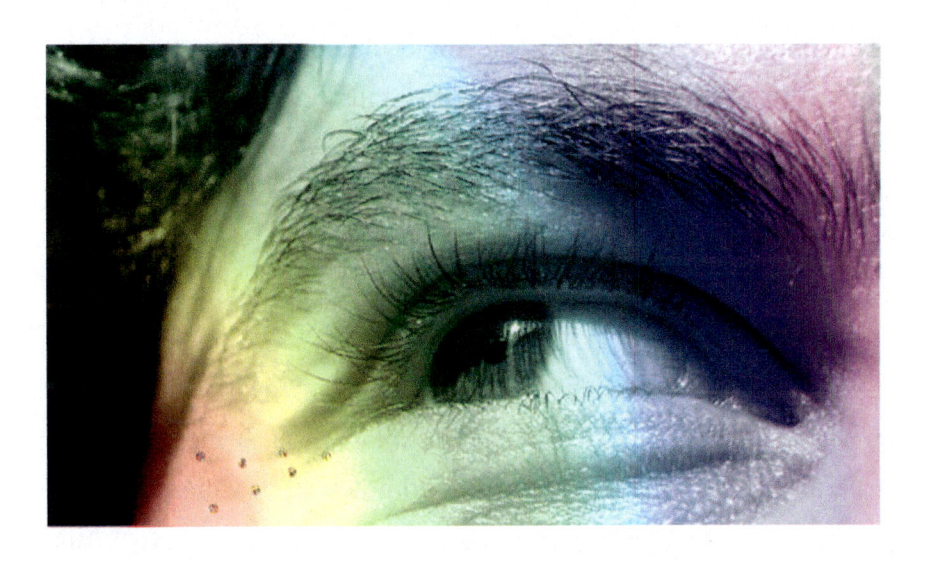

The name Floco Tausin is a pseudonym. The author received a PhD at the Faculty of the Humanities at the University of Bern, Switzerland. In theory and practice he is engaged in the research of subjective visual phenomena in connection with altered states of consciousness and the development of consciousness. In 2009, he published the mystical story Mouches Volantes about the spiritual dimension of eye floaters.

The book

Mouches Volantes. Eye Floaters as Shining Structure of Consciousness
(Spiritual Fiction. ISBN: 978-3033003378. Paperback, 15.2 x 22.9 cm / 6 x 9 inches, 368 pages).

Floco Tausin tells the story about his time of learning with spiritual teacher and seer Nestor, taking place in the hilly region of Emmental, Switzerland. The mystic teachings focus on the widely known but underestimated dots and strands floating in our field of vision, known as eye floaters or mouches volantes. Whereas in ophthalmology, floaters are considered a harmless vitreous opacity, the author gradually learns to see them and reveals the first emergence of the shining structure formed by our consciousness.

Mouches Volantes explores the topic of eye floaters in a much wider sense than the usual medical explanations. It merges scientific research, esoteric philosophy and practical consciousness development, and observes the spiritual meaning and everyday life implications of these dots and strands.

Mouches Volantes – a mystical story about the closest thing in the world.

Printed in Great Britain
by Amazon